Manual of

Clinical Dilemma in Mature Women

61st AICOG BHUBANESWAR 2018

AICOG 2018 Odisha

Manual of Clinical Dilemma in Mature Women

Editors

SN Tripathy

KC Mahapatra

SK Giri

Priya Ganesh Kumar

Jyothi Unni

Meeta

Jayshree Pattnaik

Ashok Padhi

JAYPEE *The Health Sciences Publisher*

New Delhi | London | Panama

Jaypee Brothers Medical Publishers (P) Ltd

Headquarters

Jaypee Brothers Medical Publishers (P) Ltd
4838/24, Ansari Road, Daryaganj
New Delhi 110 002, India
Phone: +91-11-43574357
Fax: +91-11-43574314
Email: jaypee@jaypeebrothers.com

Overseas Offices

J.P. Medical Ltd
83 Victoria Street, London
SW1H 0HW (UK)
Phone: +44-20 317 08910
Fax: +44 (0)20 3008 6180
Email: info@jpmedpub.com

Jaypee-Highlights Medical Publishers Inc
City of Knowledge, Bld. 235, 2nd floor, Clayton
Panama City, Panama
Phone: +1 507-301-0496
Fax: +1 507-301-0499
Email: cservice@jphmedical.com

Jaypee Brothers Medical Publishers (P) Ltd
17/1-B Babar Road, Block-B, Shyamoli
Mohammadpur, Dhaka-1207
Bangladesh
Mobile: +08801912003485
Email: jaypeedhaka@gmail.com

Jaypee Brothers Medical Publishers (P) Ltd
Bhotahity, Kathmandu, Nepal
Phone: +977-9741283608
Email: Kathmandu@jaypeebrothers.com

Website: www.jaypeebrothers.com
Website: www.jaypeedigital.com

Inquiries for bulk sales may be solicited at: jaypee@jaypeebrothers.com

Manual of Clinical Dilemma in Mature Women

First Edition: **2018**

ISBN 978-93-5270-373-9

Printed at: Samrat Offset Pvt. Ltd.

Contributors

Abraham Peedicayil
Christian Medical College and Hospital
Vellore, Tamil Nadu, India

Asaranti Kar
Srusti Hospital and Acharya Harihar Regional Cancer Centre (AHRCC)
Cuttack, Odisha, India, Lady Hardinge Medical College
New Delhi, India

Bhagyalaxmi Nayak
Srusti Hospital and Acharya Harihar Regional Cancer Centre (AHRCC)
Cuttack, Odisha, India, Lady Hardinge Medical College
New Delhi, India

Dipanwita Banerjee
Department of Gynaecological Oncology
Chittaranjan National Cancer Institute
Kolkata, West Bengal, India

Geeta Gupta
Assistant Professor
BRD Medical College
Gorakhpur, Uttar Pradesh, India

Ipsita Dhal
Srusti Hospital and Acharya Harihar Regional Cancer Centre (AHRCC)
Cuttack, Odisha, India, Lady Hardinge Medical College
New Delhi, India

Jyothi Unni

Kirubamani NH

Manisha Vernekar
Department of Gynaecological Oncology
Chittaranjan National Cancer Institute
Kolkata, West Bengal, India

Mary Ann Lumsden
Professor, Department of Gynaecology, University of Glasgow, UK
President, International Menopause Society, UK
Senior Vice President
Royal College of Obstetricians and Gynaecologists (RCOG), UK

Meeta

Niranjan Chavan
Professor and Unit Chief
Lokmanya Tilak Municipal Medical College (LTMMC)
Lokmanya Tilak Municipal General Hospital (LTMGH)
Mumbai, Maharashtra, India

Priya Ganesh Kumar

Ramani Manoj
Christian Medical College and Hospital
Vellore, Tamilnadu, India

Ramani Rajendran
Certified Colposcopist UK
Formerly Professor
Department of Obstetrics and Gynaecology
Madras Medical College
Chennai, Tamil Nadu, India

Ranajit Mandal
Department of Gynaecological Oncology
Chittaranjan National Cancer Institute
Kolkata, West Bengal, India

Ranu Patni

Rooma Sinha

Sonia Malik

Sunila Khandelwal

Tushar Kar
Srusti Hospital and Acharya Harihar Regional Cancer Centre (AHRCC)
Cuttack, Odisha, India
Lady Hardinge Medical College
New Delhi, India

Message

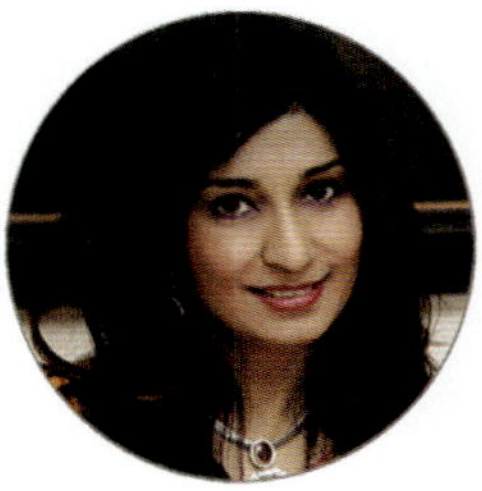

Rishma Dhillon Pai
MD DNB FCPS DGO FICOG
President, FOGSI—2017
Consultant Gynecologist
Jaslok Hospital, Lilavati Hospital and Hinduja Healthcare (Khar),
Bloom IVF Centre,
The Every Woman Clinic,
Mumbai, Maharashtra, India

"Wisdom.... comes not from age, but from education and learning."
Anton Chekhov

Life is a continuous process of learning. Especially in the field of medicine, which is constantly changing, it is very important to keep oneself abreast with the latest developments. It is heartening to note that academic workshop manuals are being released at the AICOG, Bhubaneswar, Odisha, India, for the benefit of the participating delegates and present varied updates in the field. Many different Manuals are being released on important subjects such as *3D Laparoscopy and Operative Oncology, Genetics, Fetal Medicine and Color Doppler, Postpartum Hemorrhage and High-Risk Pregnancy, Hysteroscopy,* etc.

I thank all the authors, for their immense contributions in building up the content for the manuals for Federation of Obstetric and Gynaecological Societies of India (FOGSI) by sharing their rich experiences in the field. These will be a big help to young gynecologists, who are still acquiring skills in various aspects of obstetrics and gynecology and a quick update for the seniors.

I extend congratulations to the organizing team of the AICOG 2018 and the editors of these manuals and wish you all success for this mega event.

"You cannot open a book without learning something."

—Confucius

Message

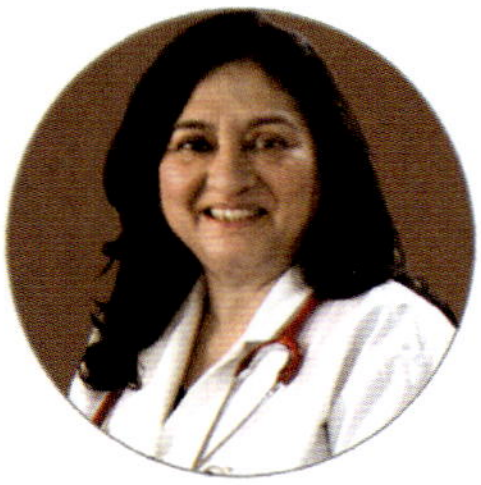

Jaideep Malhotra
MD FICMCH FICS FMAS FRCOG FICOG FRCPI FIAJAGO
Consultant ART (IVF)
President Elect, FOGSI—2018
Director, Rainbow IVF
Agra, Uttar Pradesh, India

"Education is greatest gift of life, it should never stop."

The subject of obstetrics and gynecology needs extreme proficiency as it deals with the medical specialties that focus on two different aspects. First one includes the care of pregnant women, the unborn baby, labor and delivery, as well as the immediate period following childbirth. Second aspect includes dealing with any ailment concerning the female reproductive organs. Hence, the manuals will help all those who are looking forward to gain excellence in the field of woman health. The manuals have tried to address all the issues a doctor needs.

With increasing expertise in all fields, the surgeon therefore while exercising a choice needs to follow the Hippocratic dictum—*"First, do no harm."*

We are thankful to all those who have incorporated their contribution by providing chapters from their research and collected scientific material and have shared their fruitful experiences for the delegates of the workshop.

As a part of my agenda for 2018, I as FOGSI President 2018, plan to work actively on QED (Quality, Ethics and Dignity) among our profession and also work towards HER (Health, Empowerment and Respect) towards our patients.

"Knowledge is of no value unless you put it into practices."

Message

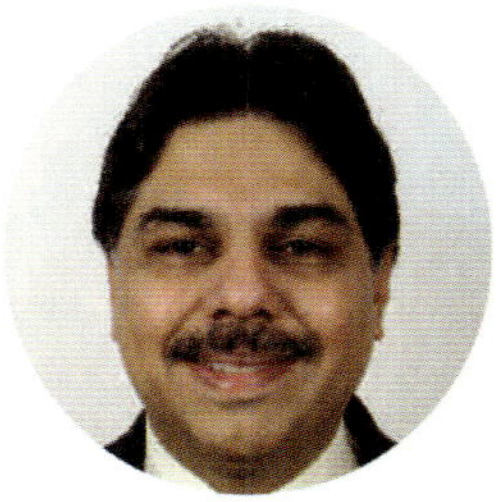

Hrishikesh Pai
Secretary General, FOGSI

It is my proud privilege to invite and welcome all delegates to the 61st All India Congress of Obstetrics and Gynaecology (AICOG) from 17th–21st January, 2018 at the Temple City of India, Bhubaneswar, Odisha, India.

It is propitious to note that the academic workshop manuals are being released which will reap beneficial reward to all the participating delegates.

I thank all the authors, for their immense contributions in building up the content for the manuals for Federation of Obstetric and Gynaecological Societies of India (FOGSI) by sharing their rich experiences in the field. These will be a big help to young gynecologists, who are still acquiring skills in various aspects of obstetrics and gynecology and a quick update for the seniors.

I forward my heartiest congratulations to all the contributors, the editors and the delegates of the workshop.

Message

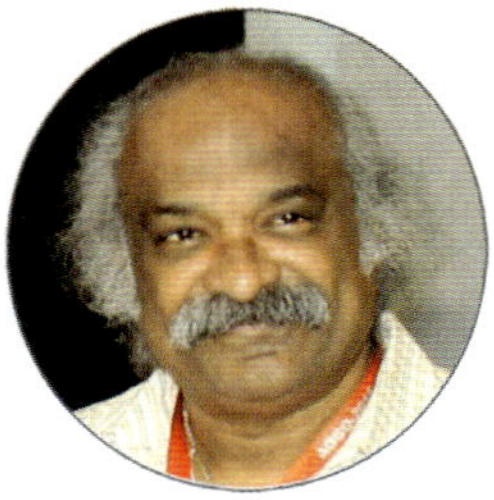

PC Mahapatra
Professor
Department of Obstetrics and Gynecology
SCB Medical College
Cuttack, Odisha, India
President, FOGSI—2011
Organising Chairperson

It is my proud privilege to invite and welcome all delegates to the 61st All India Congress of Obstetrics and Gynaecology (AICOG) from 17th–21st January, 2018 at the Temple City of India, Bhubaneswar, Odisha, India.

The five days of academic extravaganza will certainly enrich the scientific knowledge of all participating delegates and faculty. The precongress workshop on various aspects of this specialty will be held on 17th January 2018.

A quote by Edwin Louis Cole says that "*Winners are not those who never fail but those who never quit*" is apt for all the clinicians who are determined enough to see and overcome all the difficulties that are faced in the field of obstetrics and gynecology.

Today, with the advancement in the field of obstetrics and gynecology, everyone requires an in-depth knowledge of the complex subjects associated with the field so as to gain excellence in it.

This manual will prove to be a boon to all those who are associated with the field and wants to gain more knowledge in the subject matter.

Message

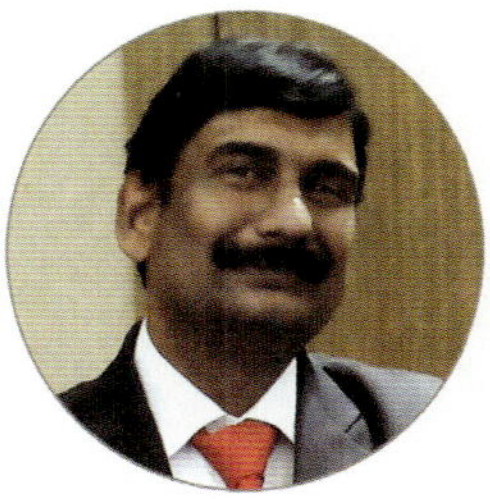

HP Pattanaik
Head
Department of Obstetrics and Gynecology
City Hospital
Cuttack, Odisha, India
Vice President, FOGSI—2009
Organising Secretary

Greetings from 61st AICOG 2018!

It is a matter of great pleasure to invite you all to 61st AICOG, from 17th–21st January, 2018 at the Temple City of India, Bhubaneswar, Odisha, India. The 11th Precongress workshops will be held on 17th January, 2018 in three medical colleges of Bhubaneswar.

It is propitious to note that the academic workshop manuals are being released which will reap beneficial reward to all the participating delegates.

It will also prove to be beneficial to the members of Federation of Obstetric and Gynaecological Societies of India (FOGSI), those who were unable to register themselves for the academic workshops.

I forward my heartiest congratulations to all the contributors, the editors and the delegates of the workshop.

Preface

What is true in science today may be the folly of tomorrow.

The field of Menopausal Medicine is constantly changing and this is now greater than ever before. It is imperative for all of us to keep pace with this change so as to enable us to give our women the best advice possible.

In this workshop on *Clinical Dilemmas in Mature Women*, we have chosen three common gynecological problems which we all encounter in our daily practice.

Polycystic ovarian syndrome is a condition which we routinely treat from adolescence and through the reproductive years, research is indicating that it has a significant impact on older women too. Metabolic issues and cancers in women with PCOS are the two main areas of concern in this age group.

Endometriosis is usually regarded as a disease of premenopause which resolves after natural or iatrogenic menopause. However, recurrence and malignant transformation can occur in later years, so prescribing hormone therapy for these women to alleviate climacteric symptoms is challenging.

There can be a significant impact of premature menopause on both physical and emotional health. Once the diagnosis has been made, several issues have to be addressed while counseling these women on the management aspects too.

Preventive oncology plays a great role in prevention of cancer, especially cervical cancer. The detection of HPV virus has changed the whole concept. HPV vaccination will go a long way in preventing cancer cervix.

In this workshop, we feel certain that listening to experts in these fields bring us the latest information and evidence that will help us feel more confident in handling these issues.

This manual is intended as a reinforcement of the deliberations of this workshop.

Knowledge is a treasure but practice is the key to it.

Editors

Contents

Chapter 1

Premature Ovarian Failure: When the Ovaries Pack Up Too Soon!

Sonia Malik

INTRODUCTION

The Indian Menopause Society recognizes an earlier age of menopause of the Indian women as compared to her Caucasian counterpart. Therefore, the age of premature menopause too would be advanced in comparison to them. Hence, according to the IMS 2015 guidelines, the age for premature menopause is less than 38 years and not 40 years.

MANAGEMENT

- Women with untreated premature menopause are at increased risk of developing osteoporosis, cardiovascular disease dementia, cognitive decline, and Parkinson's and all-cause mortality
- Counseling and lifestyle changes form the mainstay of general treatment
- Management is essentially dependent upon the requirement of the patient:
  - Fertility desired
  - Fertility not desired
  - Special conditions.

Fertility Desired

Five to ten percent of women with premature menopause can experience spontaneous resolution leading to pregnancy, although factors which could predict this outcome are not known. On the other hand, options for pregnancy are few. These are either adoption or achieving a pregnancy by oocyte or embryo donation. Oocyte donation entails preparation of the endometrium for implantation. This can be successfully achieved by incremental doses of estradiol valerate/17β estradiol from 2 to 6 mg over a 2-week period, and then progesterone therapy, which could be pessaries, 400 mg twice daily, or a vaginal gel or injectable progesterone. This creates a receptive endometrium for embryo implantation.

Pregnancy has also been reported after successful transplantation of ovarian cortex or the entire ovary, but this option is not widely available.

Fertility preservation is now possible for patients of cancer. This can be achieved by gonadal shielding, ovarian transposition, and ovarian suppression by gonadotropin-releasing hormone analogs or cryopreservation of oocyte, embryo or ovarian tissue. The suitability, timing, and success of each of these preventive interventions have been described in detail in many reviews and guidelines. In patients desirous of their own genetic children only, other options like DHEAS or testosterone gels have been advocated but their use is not yet evidence based. Others have tried estrogen suppression followed by exogenous gonadotropins. Women with premature menopause have chronically high gonadotropin levels which down-regulate follicle-stimulating hormone (FSH) receptors on granulosa cells, so that the remaining follicles become refractory to exogenous stimulation. Pretreatment with estrogens suppresses FSH serum levels and allows the restoration of FSH receptors in the remaining follicles. When this pretreatment was followed by exogenous gonadotropin stimulation, ovulation occurred in 32% of cases and among these, pregnancy was achieved in 50%.

Fertility not Desired

Contraception needs to be practiced if the woman is not desirous of a pregnancy. Barrier methods or intrauterine contraceptive devices are the preferred options. It has been suggested that oral contraceptives fail to suppress the high FSH levels characteristic of premature menopause.

Hormonal replacement therapy (HRT) forms the mainstay of management for these patients not only for VMS and vaginal symptoms but also for long-term prevention of estrogen deficient states. The indications of HRT are listed in Table 1.

Table 1 Indications for HRT use by women with POI.

Sequelae of POI	Indication for HRT?	Supporting recommendation/conclusion	Grade[1]
Vasomotor symptoms	YES	HRT is recommended	C
Genito-urinary symptoms	YES	Systemic and local estrogens are effective treatments	A
Life expectancy	?	Life expectancy appears to be reduced due to cardiovascular mortality: HRT may be of indirect benefit	n/a[2]
Bone health	YES	HRT is recommended to maintain bone health and prevent osteoporosis; it is plausible that it will reduce the risk of fracture	C
Cardiovascular health	YES	Despite lack of longitudinal outcome data, early initiation of HRT is strongly recommended to control future risk of cardiovascular disease: it should be continued until the average age of natural menopause	C
Quality of life	?	Quality of life appears to be reduced: HRT may be of indirect benefit	n/a[2]
Sexual function	YES	Adequate estrogen replacement is the starting point for normalizing sexual function. Local estrogen may also be required to treat dyspareunia	C
Neurological function	?	HRT to reduce the possible risk of cognitive impairment should be considered at least until the average age of natural menopause	C

POI, premature ovarian insufficiency; HRT, hormone replacement therapy.
[1]The grade of a recommendation reflects the strength of the evidence supporting it. Grade A indicates that the recommendation is based on a high quality systematic review or multiple randomized controlled trials (RCTs). Grade B recommendations are based on a single RCT or a large trial or study of high quality. Grade C on moderate quality trials or studies and Grade D on at least moderate quality non analytical studies.
[2]Not applicable.

Source: Adapted from European Society for Human Reproduction and Embryology (ESHRE) Guidelines for premature ovarian insufficiency (POI) 2015.

Types, Routes and Dosage

Three forms of estrogens are estradiol valerate, conjugated equine estrogens and 17β estradiol. The latter is now preferred because of its least hepatotoxic profile. Various formulations of HRT are available which can be administered by the oral, transdermal, vaginal or subcutaneous route. In the absence of any clear randomized prospective data to guide the route of administration, treatment is individualized according to choice and risk factors. In older women transdermal preparations have shown to have a decreased risk of venous thromboembolism (VTE) and CV event. A recent study has shown better cardiovascular health outcomes among women with POF who receive transdermal estradiol and vaginal progesterone compared with oral ethinylestradiol and norethisterone.

For women with a uterus, progestogen must be added as a supplement to avoid the unopposed effects of estrogen on the endometrium. Progesterone again can be prescribed as an oral or vaginal tablet depending on the choice of the patient. Evidence from older postmenopausal women favors micronized natural progesterone, as it is associated with a more favorable cardiovascular profile, and possibly reduced breast cancer risk, with similar efficacy for protecting the endometrium.

There is no data on the duration of use in these women with premature menopause.

The dose has to be titrated gradually but indicators like vasomotor symptoms may not be present in such patients. No data were identified for any particular dose for symptom relief in women with premature menopause, although transdermal 100 μg/day may be sufficient in most.

It is suggested to aim for physiological estradiol levels, as found in the serum of women with normal menstrual cycles, with an average 50–100 pg/mL (180-370 pmol/L). These levels can be achieved in women with premature menopause with 100 μg estradiol transdermally. Similar levels can be provided by 2–4 mg estradiol orally. Recent evidence suggests that 2 mg of 17β-estradiol orally is sufficient to maintain BMD (study in Turner's syndrome patients), and the effects are equal to 4 mg.

Progestogen dose depends on that the concurrent dose of estrogen and the regimen. Continuous regimens require a minimum of 1 mg of oral norethisterone daily or 2.5 mg medroxyprogesterone acetate (MPA) at the moderate to high doses of estrogen that should be provided for women with premature menopause. Sequential regimens require 10 mg MPA for a minimum of 10–12 days per month, or 200 mg oral micronized progesterone.

Monitoring

Once established on therapy, women with premature menopause using HRT should have a clinical review annually, paying particular attention to compliance. No routine monitoring tests are required but may be prompted by specific symptoms or concerns.

Special Situations

Turner's Syndrome

Girls and women with premature menopause due to Turner syndrome should be offered HRT throughout the normal reproductive lifespan.

Women with Premature Menopause and a BRCA Gene Mutation or after Breast Cancer

- Hormonal replacement therapy is generally contraindicated in breast cancer survivors.
- Hormonal replacement therapy is a treatment option for women carrying BRCA1/2 mutations but without personal history of breast cancer after prophylactic bilateral salpingo-oophorectomy (BSO).

Women with Premature Ovarian Insufficiency and Endometriosis

For women with endometriosis who required oophorectomy, combined estrogen/progestogen therapy can be effective for the treatment of vasomotor symptoms and may reduce the risk of disease reactivation.

Migraine

No studies were identified for the dose, type, or route of administration of HRT in women with POI and migraine. Data for normal postmenopausal women with migraine is also minimal and conflicting.

Migraine with aura remains a contraindication for combined oral contraceptive pill use for women with premature menopause. Transdermal delivery may be the lowest-risk route of administration of estrogen for migraine-sufferers with aura.

Hypertension

- Hypertension should not be seen as a contraindication to HRT use by women with premature menopause.
- In hypertensive women with premature menopause, transdermal estradiol is the preferred method of delivery

Venous Thromboembolism

- Women with premature menopause and a history of prior VTE or thrombophilic disorder should be referred to a hematologist prior to commencing HRT.
- Transdermal estradiol is the preferred route of delivery for women with premature menopause at increased risk of VTE.

Obesity

Transdermal estradiol is the preferred method of delivery for women with premature menopause requiring HRT who are obese or overweight.

Use of Androgens

Androgens may be required in patients who have had a surgical menopause for loss of libido. However, women should be informed that androgen treatment is only supported by limited data, and that long-term health effects are not clear yet. If androgen therapy is commenced, treatment effect should be evaluated after 3–6 months and should possibly be limited to 24 months.

The woman with premature menopause is special since she requires early intervention that continues lifelong. Since this entity has been identified recently, long-term effects of management are still unclear. The effect of this management would be clear after results of these studies start coming in.

FURTHER READING

1. ESHRE. Management of women with premature ovarian insufficiency. Guidelines of The Indian Menopause Society 2015.

Chapter 2

Etiology and Diagnosis of Premature Ovarian Insufficiency

Mary Ann Lumsden

DEFINITION

Premature ovarian insufficiency (POI) is defined as amenorrhea for 6 months and is associated with elevated follicle-stimulating hormone (FSH) and luteinizing hormone (LH) levels due to failure of the ovaries. Early menopause is when this occurs in women under 45 years of age. The prevalence is 1% of women for women under the age of 40 years, 0.1% for those under 30 and 0.01% for those under the age 20 years.[1]

The term POI is used rather than premature ovarian failure (POF) as resumption of function occurs in a small proportion of women. The exception to this is if the ovaries are absent or removed surgically.

The Physiological Process Leading to Menopause

Menopause occurs when the number of follicles in the ovary decreases below a critical level. The maximum number of follicles is present in the ovary during fetal life and decreases consistently with an accelerated rate of decline as menopause approaches. It is this rate of decline which determines the age of menopause, occurring earlier in those who subsequently go through premature menopause.

DIAGNOSIS

This is covered in the Guideline 'Menopause: Diagnosis and Management' published by the National Institute of Health and Care Excellence (NICE in 2015).[2] The diagnosis is covered in the recommendations included in the Box 1.

Following these recommendations is important in order to distinguish the cause of the secondary amenorrhea from other causes of such as hypogonadotropic hypogonadism or polycystic ovarian syndrome:

Box 1: NICE Guideline 2015: Menopause: Diagnosis and Management

11.1.8: Recommendations

53. Take into account the woman's clinical history (for example, previous medical or surgical treatment) and family history when diagnosing premature ovarian insufficiency

54. Diagnose premature ovarian insufficiency in women aged under 40 years based on:

- Menopausal symptoms, including no or infrequent periods (taking into account whether the woman has a uterus) and
- Elevated FSH levels on 2 blood samples taken 4–6 weeks apart

55. Do not diagnose premature ovarian insufficiency on the basis of a single blood test

56. Do not routinely use anti-Müllerian hormone testing to diagnose premature ovarian insufficiency

57. If there is doubt about the diagnosis of premature ovarian insufficiency, consider anti-Müllerian hormone testing after seeking specialist advice (see the NICE guideline on fertility)[3]

- No periods/irregular periods for 4 months
- FSH X 2 (>25 IU/L) >6 weeks apart
- Low estradiol.

Other things that can be measured and may help lead to a diagnosis are anti-Müllerian hormone (AMH), antral follicle count and inhibin, although as far as diagnosis goes, FSH is likely to be sufficient.

ETIOLOGY

The etiology includes following:

Genetic[4]

There are some disorders that are more commonly associated with POI. Turner's syndrome or mosaic may present with secondary amenorrhea and subfertility as may Fragile X disease. The latter is important as it may be associated with mental retardation and counseling of family members is therefore of importance.

The majority of women affected by familial POI (FPOI) do not know the genetic cause of their disease and so counseling of their family members (daughters, sisters, nieces, cousins) about the chances of developing the disease is impossible although maternal age is the single most important factor in predicting menopausal age. Furthermore, there is currently no test available to predict this disease, and for most women, the condition is diagnosed when their menstrual pattern changes or menstruation ceases; a time when it is too late to achieve a pregnancy. Moreover, there is no treatment available to reverse, suspend or slow the abnormal ovarian function due to limited research and access to genetic analysis.

Familial, twin, population and targeted gene approach studies have shown that genetic abnormalities play a significant and major role in idiopathic POI, with only a minimal contribution from environmental causes. At least 30% of idiopathic POI cases run in families (familial POI; FPOI) and this percentage is likely to be higher because of a reduced capacity for affected women to transmit the condition to her children. FPOI is likely to be the result of a number of Mendelian disorders and represents a distinct cause of POI and familial studies suggest that early onset disease is more likely to be associated with highly penetrant mutations. This Mendelian pattern has been confirmed in a small number of pedigrees studied in detail, there mutations in a number of genes. Therefore, the existence of a myriad of, as yet undiscovered, genetic aberrations contributing to FPOI is a certainty.

Iatrogenic

Surgical removal: Bilateral oophorectomy is undertaken at hysterectomy undertaken to treat estrogen dependent disease such as endometriosis. They may also be removed in those with a high incidence of hormone dependent cancer, e.g. in women who have *BRCA1/2* gene mutations. Oophorectomy was a standard procedure for women following breast cancer in the past although medical treatments are now more commonly used.

Cytotoxic treatments, e.g. medical or radiological treatments for cancer can cause ovarian failure because of they destroy rapidly dividing cells in the ovaries and depleting the supply of oocytes. The chance of ovarian function resuming depends on the cytotoxic regimen used and the age of the patients. This is particularly true for hematological cancers where the change of survival has increased dramatically and is common in young women.

Autoimmune Disorders

Autoantibodies may be found and POI can also be associated with deficiencies in other glands such as thyroid and so thyroid function tests might be required.

Environmental Toxins

Smoking is well known to lead to early ovarian failure.

CONSEQUENCES

Premature ovarian insufficiency impacts on the following areas of health.

Cognitive Impairment

Premenopausal oophorectomized women are at increased risk of cognitive impairment[5] and Parkinsonism.[6] The risk is increased with younger age at oophorectomy and there is a protective role for estrogen replacement.

In a French cohort study of 4868 women, both spontaneous and iatrogenic POI were associated with negative effects on cognitive function in later life.[7] There is an increased risk of poor verbal fluency and visual memory. The UK Biobank data that studied women with POI identified that the use of HRT was associated with improved markers of cognitive function.[8]

Osteoporosis

Women with POI have significantly lower bone density compared to controls and increased fracture risk.[9] There is also evidence that HRT use for more than 3 years may reduce fracture risk.[10] For every unit increase in time (month) BMD as measured by spine T score decrease by 0.026, $p = 0.001$ (1 way anova).[11]

Life Expectancy

Mean life expectancy in POI is 2 years less than menopause at over 55 years. This decrease may be for a number of reasons including a higher incidence of cardiovascular disease.[12]

Cardiovascular Disease

There is an 80% increased risk of mortality from ischemic heart disease in POI compared to those with menopause at 49–55 years.[13] Ischemic heart disease mortality is increased for those with early age at natural menopause compared with those with normal age at natural menopause.[14]

The risk is more pronounced in those who have never used estrogens. The reasons for this alteration in CVD risk include impaired endothelial function, adverse effects on the lipid profile, reduced insulin sensitivity and increased metabolic syndrome. Women with POI should be advised to reduce cardiovascular risk factors by not smoking, taking regular exercise and maintaining a healthy weight. Fatal and nonfatal total cardiovascular disease is increased in POI.[15]

Depression

The reasons for an increased chance of depression is multi-factorial but is likely to include loss of fertility for many of the affected women particularly in those under 30 years and those diagnosed in infertility clinics.

The hormone changes of the perimenopause may also be conducive to development of depression and low mood as occurs at the time of the natural menopause.

Sexual Dysfunction

Superficial dyspareunia and vulvovaginal atrophy can occur because of the lack of estrogen and respond well to administration of local estrogen. Other causes will include loss of fertility and a change in self-perception and self-image.

Fertility

This will be a subject of a separate presentation at this meeting.

REFERENCES

1. Coulam CB, Adamson SC, Annegers JF. Incidence of premature ovarian failure. Obstet Gynecol. 1986;67(4):604-6.
2. NICE Guideline No. 23.
3. NICE Guideline Fertility problems: assessment and treatment (CG156) 2013 updated 2017.
4. Chapman et al. The genetics of Premature Ovarian Failure. Int J Women's Health. 2015;7:799-810.
5. Rocca WA, Gazzuola Rocca L, Smith CY, et al. Bilateral Oophorectomy and Accelerated Aging: Cause or Effect? J Gerontol A Biol Sci Med Sci. 2017;72(9):1213-7.
6. Rocca WA, Grossardt BR, Geda YE, et al. Long-term risk of depressive and anxiety symptoms after early bilateral oophorectomy. Menopause. 2008;15(6):1050-9.
7. Soni M, Hogervorst E. Premature ovarian insufficiency and neurological function. Minerva Endocrinol. 2014;39(3):189-99. Epub 2014 Jun 19. Review.
8. Iliodromiti. Oral presentation International Menopause Society Meeting Prague; 2016.
9. van Der Voort DJ, van Der Weijer PH, Barentsen R. Early menopause: increased fracture risk at older age Osteoporos Int. 2003;14(6):525-30. Epub 2003 Apr 30.
10. van der Klift M1, de Laet CE, McCloskey EV, et al. Risk factors for incident vertebral fractures in men and women: the Rotterdam Study. J Bone Miner Res. 2004;19(7):1172-80. Epub 2004 Feb 23.
11. Panay N, Maclaran K, Shah G, et al. 2017; https://poiregsitry.net
12. Ossewaarde ME, Bots ML, Verbeek AL, et al. Age at menopause, cause-specific mortality and total life expectancy. Epidemiology. 2005;16(4):556-62.
13. Tao X-Y, Zuo A-Z, Wang FB, et al. Effect of primary ovarian insufficiency and early natural menopause on mortality: A meta-analysis. Climacteric. 2016;19:27-36.
14. Jacobsen BK, Knutsen SF, Fraser GE. Age at natural menopause and total mortality and mortality from ischemic heart disease: the Adventist Health Study J Clin Epidemiol. 1999;52(4):303-7.
15. Daan NM, Muka T, Koster MP, et al. Cardiovascular Risk in Women With Premature Ovarian Insufficiency Compared to Premenopausal Women at Middle Age. J Clin Endocrinol Metab. 2016;101(9):3306-15. doi: 10.1210/jc.2016-1141. Epub 2016 Jun 14.

Chapter 3

How Ominous is Polycystic Ovary Syndrome at Menopause?

Kirubamani NH

It is not possible to diagnose a woman with polycystic ovary syndrome (PCOS) when she has already reached menopause because the cardinal features disappear. While the research on menopausal/PCOS mechanisms is sparse, we do know that because PCOS affects many of the body's systems, the responses of each of these systems to aging will vary and they will also vary according to the individual. PCOS is a lifelong disease. It is a challenge to distinguish menopausal changes from abnormalities connected with PCOS. The expression of PCOS may begin early and the symptoms change across the lifespan. Determining the appearance and expression of the syndrome at each stage of life will be important to expand the diagnosis and treatment of PCOS.

Polycystic ovary syndrome in postmenopausal women is not well-defined as there is no robust criteria. Regarding PCOS at menopause a few questions that cross our mind are:

- Does PCOS get worse and if so, how worse?
- Does PCOS get better after menopause?
- Could PCOS simply disappear altogether?

Criteria for the Metabolic Syndrome according to the National Cholesterol Education Program (NCEP), Adult Treatment Panel III

Three or more of the following:

- Elevated waist circumference—greater than 35 inches (88 cm)
- Elevated triglycerides—equal to or greater than 150 mg/dL
- High-density lipoprotein (HDL)—less than 50 mg/dL
- Elevated blood pressure—equal to or greater than 130/85 mm Hg
- Elevated fasting glucose—equal to or greater than 100 mg/dL.

Hyperandrogenism seen in PCOS women persists after the menopausal transition. Similarly, PCOS women continue to manifest the metabolic alterations such as insulin resistance after menopause, which makes them more susceptible to type 2 diabetes mellitus.

Older women with PCOS still had lower levels of sex hormone binding globulin (SHBG). Postmenopausal women with PCOS are exposed to higher adrenal and ovarian androgen levels than non-PCOS women. The metabolic features are primarily related to underlying insulin resistance (IR), which is now understood to play an important role in both the pathogenesis and long-term sequelae of PCOS. The data published by Puurunen et al. revealed that enhanced ovarian androgen secretion along with unfavorable metabolic changes such as impaired glucose tolerance, chronic inflammation which were observed in a group of premenopausal women with PCOS, persist after the menopausal transition. The prevalence of hypertension was higher in postmenopausal women with PCOS compared with controls studied longitudinally, and triglyceride levels increased in both groups but remained higher in the women with PCOS. Livadas S. et al found that insulin resistance was positively associated with body mass index (BMI) and androgens level. Lean females with PCOS may present a better metabolic profile with time and PCOS may even remain as a silent disorder. It is possible that the metabolic abnormalities in women with PCOS worsen with age, because all women experience increasing insulin resistance and abdominal adiposity along with chronic inflammation and dyslipidemia with age and a specific increase in LDL across the menopausal transition. These events are partially related to persisting hyperandrogenism but are mostly correlated with excessive body weight (mainly visceral obesity). This suggests that our best long-term strategy is to ensure that women with PCOS are informed about their high-risk for metabolic and cardiovascular diseases. Women who remained anovulatory, with aging had increases in total cholesterol, low-density lipoprotein (LDL), HDL levels reduced and cardiovascular risk remained significantly higher than in the general population according to Carmina E, Campagna A, et al. Although there was an increased prevalence of type 2 diabetes in women with PCOS, compared with controls at a younger age; the prevalence of type 2 diabetes increased with age in controls, and there was no difference in the prevalence of diabetes 20 years later when women with PCOS had reached menopause. There was also no difference in fasting insulin levels, homeostatic model assessment (HOMA) of insulin resistance, and glucose levels in the two groups at an older age according to Schmidt J, Brännström M, et al. The suggestion of various studies is that "if women with PCOS do not become obese they may exhibit a better metabolic profile. The long-term risk for morbidity and mortality among postmenopausal women with a history of PCOS is uncertain and there is no established phenotype for PCOS after menopause. Long-term, multicenter cohort studies are needed where the following issues should be assessed: menopausal phenotype, metabolic syndrome, cardiovascular events, and other causes of morbidity/mortality. Small numbers of studies during menopause, point to the need for additional longitudinal studies to expand the current knowledge. The ongoing studies will provide a thorough understanding of the PCOS lifecycle, to help with diagnosis and treatment that is no longer limited to the reproductive-age patient and should extent to menopausal women. PCOS must be managed throughout a woman's life and dietary and lifestyle changes can improve their health and lower their risk of chronic disease.

Polycystic ovary syndrome at menopause will be "ominous" when the woman increases her abdominal circumferences and BMI.

Chapter 4

PCOS and Cancers at Menopause

Ranu Patni

INTRODUCTION

Polycystic ovary syndrome (PCOS) begins in majority of cases at the perimenarcheal period or before bone age reaches 16 years. However, it may go clinically unrecognized till a much later age due to ignorance of symptoms like irregular menstruation, hirsutism, etc. In lean women with a genetic predisposition to PCOS, the syndrome may be unmasked when they subsequently gain weight.[1] PCOS occurs due to abnormal metabolism of androgens and estrogen along with abnormality in control of androgen production. High serum concentrations of testosterone, androstenedione and dehydroepiandrosterone sulfate (DHEA-S) may be found in these patients. At the same time, there are individual variations and some patients have normal androgen levels also. Peripheral insulin resistance and hyperinsulinemia are also associated with PCOS. Obesity amplifies the degree of both these abnormalities.

According to the guidelines given in November 2015 by American Association of Clinical Endocrinologists (AACE), American College of Endocrinology (ACE) and Androgen Excess and PCOS Society (AES) the diagnostic criteria for PCOS should include two of the following three criteria:

1. Chronic anovulation
2. Hyperandrogenism (clinical/biologic)
3. Polycystic ovaries.

Currently, there are no diagnostic criteria for PCOS in perimenopausal or menopausal woman; however, clinicians often make a reasonable diagnosis based upon a history of prior oligomenorrhea and hyperandrogenism.[2] PCOS can persist during perimenopausal and postmenopausal periods. It is not relieved or cured by menopause.

In PCOS, there are numerous potential mechanisms which could promote malignant disease including the prolonged anovulatory status and associated imbalance between androgen and estrogen action, insulin resistance and secondary hyperinsulinemia.[3] It is a well-known fact that the risk of malignancy increases with age. The coexistence of PCOS and menopause can, therefore, lead to an increased risk of cancer. Hence, it is very essential that this condition should be recognized and managed around and after menopause.

Patients with PCOS are at an increased risk for endometrial hyperplasia and carcinoma.[4] Studies have noted a 2.7-fold increased risk for developing endometrial cancer versus general population.[5] The chronic anovulation in PCOS leads to constant endometrial stimulation with estrogen without progesterone, and this increases the risk of endometrial hyperplasia and carcinoma.[6] No known association with breast or ovarian cancer has been found, thus, no additional surveillance is needed.[6]

Barry et al. performed a systematic review and meta-analysis of observational studies and concluded that women of all ages with PCOS are at increased risk of endometrial cancer.[7] The obtained data failed to confirm the increased risk of ovarian and breast cancer in PCOS patients.[7] PCOS women are not more likely to develop breast cancer, controlling for obesity. There are insufficient data to link PCOS with vaginal, vulvar and cervical cancer.

More research is required to precisely define the overall cancer risk in PCOS population. However, current data indicate that in women with PCOS there is a significant cancer risk, at least for the endometrium. This finding should facilitate proper screening strategies, lifestyle changes and metformin treatment as a primary intervention what may decrease the risk in PCOS population.[8]

REFERENCES

1. Barber TM, Wass JA, Franks S, et al. Obesity and polycystic ovary syndrome. Clin Endocrinol (Oxf). 2006;65:137-45.
2. Puuruuen J, Piltonen T, Morin-Papunen L, et al. Unfavorable hormonal, metabolic, and inflammatory alterations persist after menopause in women with PCOS. J Clin Endocrinol Metab. 2011;96(6):1827-34.
3. Boyd DB. Insulin and cancer. Integr Cancer Ther. 2003;2:315-29.
4. Hardiman P, Pillay OC, Antonio W. Polycystic ovary syndrome and endometrial carcinoma. Lancet. 2003;361(9371):1810-2.
5. Haoula Z, Salman M, Atiomo W. Evaluating the association between endometrial cancer and polycystic ovary syndrome. Hum Reprod. 2012;27(5):1327-31.
6. RCOG. Long-term consequences of polycystic ovary syndrome. London. UK: Royal College of Obstetricians and Gynaecologists; 2007.
7. Barry JA, Azizia MM, Hardiman PJ. Risk of endometrial, ovarian and breast cancer in women with polycystic ovary syndrome: a systematic review and meta-analysis. Hum Reprod Update. 2014;20:748-58.
8. Levart-Lipinska M, Matyjaszek-Matuszek B, Woźniakowskaet E, al. Polycystic ovary syndrome: clinical implication in perimenopause. Prz Menopauzalny. 2014;13(6):348-51.

Chapter 5

And It Came Back Yet Again: Medical Aspects of Postmenopausal Endometriosis

Sunila Khandelwal

INTRODUCTION

Endometriosis is a common chronic benign gynecological disease affecting about 6–10% of all women. It is characterized by the presence of endometrium-like tissue outside the uterine cavity, primarily on the ovaries and is an estrogen-dependent condition generally limited to reproductive age. It progresses mostly in cases of moderate and severe disease but spontaneous regression can occur in 58% of milder cases. In most cases, symptoms will improve after the natural menopause or a surgical menopause but often relapses after surgical therapy, while medical therapy leads symptoms of estrogen deprivation, which has great impact on a woman's life.

Natural history is still uncharted to a large extent. This heterogeneous disease with an unpredictable evolution also affect postmenopausal women (2–5%), has comorbidity and iatrogenic consequences. Endometriosis once established can persist in the presence of low circulating levels of estrogen as seen in the postmenopausal period. Local estradiol production by the endometriotic lesions drives the disease through autocrine and paracrine effects. If endometriosis does occur in the postmenopausal period, it is less common, is present in smaller volumes and is less active. Yet, it has the same immunochemical profile as the disease occurring in premenopausal women and has the potential to reactivate when given the appropriate stimulation. Endometriosis is associated with an increased risk of epithelial ovarian cancer.[1] Unopposed estrogen therapy may play a role in the development of such tumors.

The purpose of medical and conservative surgical treatment of endometriosis is often to relieve symptoms in anticipation of a naturally occurring menopause. Occasionally, it is necessary to perform radical surgery with hysterectomy and bilateral oophorectomy to control symptoms and to avoid further surgery. An early menopause or severe menopausal complaints raise a new problem concerning hormone therapy (HT) in this group of patients.

Use of menopausal hormone treatment in women with prior history of endometriosis raises concerns in the mind of clinicians about disease recurrence with pain symptoms, need for surgery and possibly malignant transformation of residual endometriosis.

Based on literature review, consensus of expert opinion and updated researches, learning objective is to answer the queries related to:

- Is treatment always required?
- Who needs treatment?
- What kind of treatment?
- Does any treatment really work?

This presentation will highlight evidence-based practical recommendations on clinical issues:

- Is it prudent to offer HT?
- What are the risks?
- What type of HT should be given and when should treatment be initiated?
- What alternatives to HT should be proposed?
- How should these women be followed up?

The data regarding menopausal hormone therapy (MHT) regimens are limited in endometriosis patient after menopause. Estrogen-based HT is required in women with premature or early menopause until the average age of the natural menopause and should be considered in older women with severe climacteric symptoms. Various position statements on the management of the menopause in women, with a past history of endometriosis, suggested that it may be safer to give either continuous combined estrogen–progestogen therapies or tibolone in both hysterectomised and nonhysterectomised women as the risk of recurrence may be reduced.[2] Using progestogens for longer periods to treat endometriosis, the possibility of increased breast cancer risk and clinical benefits have to be weighed. As per randomized controlled trials, micronized progesterone and dydrogesterone [Continuous combined estrogen–progestogen therapy (CCEPRT)-estradiol 1 mg + dydrogesterone 5 mg/day] when used as postmenopausal HT seem to have a safer risk profile on the breast.[3]

TREATMENT

Treatment options for postmenopausal endometriosis:

- *Surgical:* First-line treatment or treatment of choice
  - Any postmenopausal mass has a potential risk of malignancy, therefore, to be removed.
- *Medical:* Second line or as an alternate first line.
  - Risk of malignant transformation of endometriosis and recurrence rates after surgery are increased.
  - Whenever surgery is contradicted.

  Aim is to alter the hormonal pathway leading to endometriosis progress.

Agents

- Gonadotropin-releasing hormone agonists (leuprorelin acetate, buserelin acetate and triptorelin)
- Combined oral contraceptives, currently, is one of the first choice for symptomatic medical therapies. At menopause CCEPRT or ultra-low-dose MHT (ethinyl estradiol/estradiol valerate + progestins).
- Tibolone
- *Progestins:* First-line therapy [Norethisterone acetate (NETA), medroxyprogesterone acetate (MPA), drospirenone, levonorgestrel-releasing intrauterine device (LNG-IUD), dydrogesterone and dienogest].
- *Aromatase inhibitors (AIs):* Letrozole and anastrozole.
- *Selective progesterone receptor modulators (SPRMs):* Ulipristal acetate (UA).

Data regarding testosterone addition are lacking in women with endometriosis.

Active postmenopausal endometriosis may be treated surgically or pharmacologically. Aromatase inhibitors may improve symptoms and treat these patients, either as first-line treatment, when surgery is contraindicated or as a second line for recurrences following surgical treatment. AIs and newer progestins (Dienogest) are emerging as promising treatment options. UA is an SPRM (effective emergency contraceptive) and has a high affinity for progesterone receptors A and B and less affinity for the glucocorticoid receptor as compared to mifepristone. In women programmed for surgical treatment for uterine fibroids with or without adenomyosis, oral UA treatment (5 or 10 mg/day) controls symptoms, reduces tumor size and improves quality of life as compared to placebo and is not inferior to monthly intramuscular injection of leuprolide acetate for 3 months. Clinical outcomes of UA treatment should be compared with surgical and other nonsurgical interventions.

FOLLOW-UP

Regular follow-up is recommended to ascertain recurrence of symptoms and adjust HT regimens. This is especially important in women with residual disease. Management of potential recurrence is best monitored by responding to recurrence of symptoms. If symptoms recur, HT should be stopped and the pain investigated. There are no sensitive markers for the diagnosis of endometriosis, except for diagnostic laparoscopy, which is gold standard. Women not wanting estrogen or those who are advised against should be offered alternative pharmacological treatment for climacteric symptoms or skeletal protection if indicated. Herbal preparations should be avoided as their efficacy is uncertain and some may contain estrogenic compounds.

Multicenter randomized trials or large observational studies are urgently needed to inform clinicians and patients alike.

KEY MESSAGES[4]

- Be aware of a possible risk for malignant transformation (although the incidence is likely to be very small).
- Advise the patient to seek medical attention if she experiences endometriosis like symptoms, especially if she is using MHT.
- Evaluate the benefits and risks of MHT for the individual patient, considering age, previous disease severity, family history, comorbidities, and body mass index.
- Actively engage the patient in the decision-making process and understand our limitation as providers to quantify specific risks.
- If the decision to initiate or continue MHT is made, consider choosing a combined hormone replacement therapy (HRT) preparation instead of an estrogen-only formulation, taking into consideration the increased risk of breast cancer with combined HRT.
- Consider alternative therapies [e.g. tibolone, aromatase inhibitors, dienogest, selective estrogen receptor modulators (SERMs) combined with estrogens].
- Consider obtaining tissue for histology if any suspicion of malignancy.

For women with a history of endometriosis who undergo surgical menopause, clinicians must balance the benefits of HRT to bone and cardiovascular health against the potential risks of recurrence or malignancy. The decision when to initiate HRT must be individualized, considering her age and past medical history.

FUTURE RESEARCH

There are many promising areas for future research in this group of women. Search retrieved no papers on the use of alternative SERMs in postmenopausal patients with history of endometriosis. There are some studies testing the gynecologic safety of SERMs, such as ospemifene and bazedoxifene, and combining these agents with estrogens (especially bazedoxifene/conjugated estrogens).[5] Such studies have been promising, and may represent a future alternative to conventional HRT.

As per American Society for Reproductive Medicine, "endometriosis should be viewed as a chronic disease that requires a lifelong management plan with the goal of maximizing the use of medical treatment and avoiding repeated surgical procedures."

Rehabilitation clinics for endometriosis patients, aimed at maintaining their physical fitness and providing psychological care, should be available and accessible.

REFERENCES

1. Rozenberg S1, Antoine C, Vandromme J, et al. Should we abstain from treating women with endometriosis using menopausal hormone therapy, for fear of an increased ovarian cancer risk? Climacteric. 2015;18(4):448-52.

2. Dunselman GA, Vermeulen N, Becker C, et al. ESHRE guideline: management of women with endometriosis. Hum Reprod. 2014;29:400-12.
3. Chlebowski RT, Rohan TE, Manson JE, et al. Breast cancer after use of estrogen plus progestin and estrogen alone: analyses of data from 2 women's health initiative randomized clinical trials. JAMA Oncol. 2015;1:296-305.
4. Gemmell LC, Webster KE, Kirtley S, et al. The Management of menopause in women with a history of endometriosis: a systematic review. Hum Reprod Update. 2017;23(4):481-509.
5. Mirkin S, Pinkerton JV, Kagan R, et al. Gynecologic safety of conjugated estrogens plus bazedoxifene: pooled analysis of five phase 3 trials. J Womens Health (Larchmt). 2016;25:431-42.

Chapter 6

And It Comes Back Yet Again: Postmenopausal Endometriosis Surgical Aspects

Rooma Sinha

INTRODUCTION

Endometriosis is a progressive problem throughout life and menopausal status is no exception although rare. Postmenopausal endometriosis was first reported in 1950. It should be considered in women in postmenopausal age group, who present with classical symptoms of endometriosis, mostly pain. In women with surgical menopause, there is a 15% probability of persistent pain after hysterectomy for endometriosis and a 3–5% risk of worsening pain or new symptom development. In fact, 2–5% of postmenopausal women have endometriosis and symptoms can recur even after decades.

When estrogen levels are low in menopause, it may prevent new lesions of endometriosis from developing, but it would not do anything to the existing lesions and the pain caused by them.

REASONS FOR THIS PROBLEM

- Estradiol production is reduced by the ovary, but estrone is produced in other areas of the body.
- Endometriosis tissue itself produces estrogen, thus promoting its own growth through autocrine and paracrine effects.
- Adhesions due to endometriosis develop into scars involving organs and nerves. The old or burnt out scars are biologically very active, invading into rectum and ureter and continue to respond to changes in circulating hormone levels.

MENOPAUSE AND ENDOMETRIOSIS—THREE SCENARIOS

1. Surgical menopause—resurgence of endometriosis
2. Known case of endometriosis—no surgery and symptomatic in menopause
3. Unknown case but symptoms and signs suggestive of endometriosis.

Surgical Menopause—Resurgence of Endometriosis

Hysterectomy is an ablative method, known to be effective in pain relief associated with endometriosis. When initial surgery is done for endometriosis, it is recommended to remove uterus along with bilateral ovaries.[1] Despite this, it does not guarantee to cure the disease completely and there is the risk of recurrence. During surgery, one or both ovaries are left behind either due to patient's desire or as a surgical team's decision. Even if both ovaries have been removed, there may be some endometrial tissue left behind attached to other organs that will now need to be addressed by surgery. Ovarian conservation carries a sixfold risk of recurrent pain and eightfold risk of reoperation. The recurrence and pelvic pain are directly correlated to the surgical precision and removal of peritoneal and deeply infiltrated disease. One must try to eradicate all endometriotic lesions to reduce the risk of recurrence.

Known Case of Endometriosis—No Surgery Done and Symptomatic in Menopause

In this category, most patients have had medical management. Medical therapy is chosen because either the disease was minimal to moderate or the patient did not desire surgery. This group will often be the one who had fertility issues. Surgical clearance of endometriosis in this group during menopause will not only relieve their symptoms but will also confirm the diagnosis. Most ovarian endometriomas are benign; however, there is a growing area of evidence regarding the relationship between endometriosis and ovarian cancer. It will be assuring to know that the complex mass seen on imaging is not malignant and confirmed by histopathology. The risk of malignant transformation of endometriosis deposits is higher in postmenopausal women especially in women with long-standing history of ovarian endometriosis.[2,3]

Unknown Case but Symptoms and Signs Suggestive of Endometriosis

This is the group of patients who are not aware that they have endometriosis. They are usually symptomatic with dysmenorrhea and there may be some subfertility issues. Managed medically with medications, succeeded and waited for menopause to finally relieve them of symptoms. They often use hormone therapy for symptomatic relief and if estrogen alone was used this may be one of the causative factors for resurgence of the problem at menopause. The hormones increase endometriosis as the density of estrogen receptors in endometriotic tissue appears to be unchanged in older patients. Even phytoestrogens have been known to exert estrogenic effects on the uterus, breast, and pituitary and support growth of endometriotic deposits.[4,5]

SURGICAL ASPECTS

Surgery is the first choice of treatment in women with postmenopausal endometriosis mainly due to the risk of malignancy. The lesions need to be surgically excised by a skilled surgeon by minimally access surgery. Laparoscopic treatment improves pain symptoms in these women. In a larger series, Redwine[6] was able to excise completely all residual endometriosis laparoscopically in 61% of 75 women with previous hysterectomy and bilateral oophorectomy, with the remainder requiring laparotomy. He noted significant improvements in pain scores after this treatment. Robotic surgery with its advantages reduces the conversion to laparotomy. However, surgery in such patients may carry some risks. Firstly, these women may have comorbidities. Secondly, many of these patients may have dense adhesion leading to higher operative risks. Nevertheless, surgery should be considered, explained, and offered to these patients.

Good preoperative imaging and bowel preparation before the procedure, including a low residue diet, will help to achieve the desired surgical results. High suspicion for deep infiltrating or obstructing lesions is useful in planning the surgery and getting a multidisciplinary team for optimal outcome.

Laparoscopic excision should be performed using scissors for sharp dissection using monopolar electrocautery. All visible endometriosis should be removed. Robotic-assisted laparoscopy is the game changer in the visualization and excision of lesions. This enables precise and meticulous resection of all endometriotic implants including deep infiltrating endometriosis. Bowel and ovarian adhesions are seen frequently in cases after hysterectomy performed for pelvic endometriosis. Laparotomy, partial, full-thickness or segmental bowel resections may be needed. Ureteric stenting may be necessary or cystoscopy performed at the completion of surgery to show bilateral ureteric patency. Colorectal patency can be performed by injection of methylene blue via a large Foley catheter placed in the lower rectum.

REFERENCES

1. Edmonds DK. Endometriosis. In: Whitfield CR (Ed). Dewhurst's Textbook of Obstetrics and Gynaecology for Postgraduates. Oxford: Blackwell Science; 1995. p. 577.
2. Cumiskey J, Whyte P, Kelehan P, et al. A detailed morphologic and immunohistochemical comparison of pre- and postmenopausal endometriosis. J Clin Pathol. 2008;61(4):455-9.
3. Brinton LA, Gridley G, Persson I, et al. Cancer risk after a hospital discharge diagnosis of endometriosis. Am J Obstet Gynecol. 1997;176(3):572-9.
4. Rattanachaiyanont M, Tanmahasamut P, Angsuwatthana S, et al. Hormonal replacement therapy in surgical menopause with underlying endometriosis. J Med Assoc Thai. 2003;86(8):702-7.
5. Cotroneo MS, Lamartiniere CA. Pharmacologic, but not dietary, genistein supports endometriosis in a rat model. Toxicol Sci. 2001;61(1):68-75.
6. Redwine DB. Laparoscopic en bloc resection for treatment of the obliterated cul-de-sac in endometriosis. J Reprod Med. 1992;37(8):695-8.

Chapter 7

Summary of Guidelines on Premature Menopause, Endometriosis and Polycystic Ovarian Disease

Meeta, Jyothi Unni

INTRODUCTION

Decisions about hormone therapy should be based on the unique health benefits and risks of the woman, age or time from menopause, and goals of therapy. The following recommendations are from guidelines on menopausal health from different organizations on premature menopause, endometriosis and polycystic ovarian disease (PCOD).

PREMATURE MENOPAUSE

- Premature ovarian insufficiency (POI) (also known as premature menopause) is defined as primary hypogonadism before the age of 40 years in women with a normal karyotype who previously had normal menstrual cycles.
- POI is the spontaneous menopause occurring 2 standard deviations (SDs) below the mean estimated age for the reference population. Traditionally, it is considered to be below the age of 40 years. In India, we may consider it as occurring below the age of 38 years.
- Women with POI have health risks that may include persistent vasomotor symptoms, genitourinary syndrome, bone loss, mood changes, and increased risk of heart disease, dementia, stroke, Parkinson disease, ophthalmic disorders, and overall mortality.
- The diagnosis of POI is confirmed by the finding of follicular stimulating hormone (FSH) levels 40 IU/l on two occasions 4–6 weeks apart. Investigation of POI should include hormone analysis, screening for autoimmune causes, karyotyping, fragile X premutation testing, pelvic, and breast ultrasound, dual X-ray absorptiometry (optional).
- It is important to inform the woman of the diagnosis with empathy in a sensitive and caring manner. Appropriate counseling, lifestyle modification

and hormone therapy (HT) form the mainstay of treatment. HT should be started as early as possible in women with POI and continued till age of natural menopause. Androgen replacement should be considered for women with persistent fatigue, loss of libido in spite of estrogen replacement.

- POI should be effectively treated to prevent an increase in the risk of cardiovascular disease, osteoporosis, cognitive decline, dementia and Parkinsonism. Observational data suggest that benefits exceed the risks for effects on prevention of osteoporosis and fracture, CVD, cognition and mood concerns, genitourinary syndrome of menopause, sexual function, and Parkinson disease longer lifespan, and reduced risk of dementia require confirmation in RCTs.
- In contrast to the treatment of postmenopausal osteopenia or osteoporosis, which focuses on bisphosphonates as first-line therapy, low bone mass in women with primary ovarian insufficiency is managed most appropriately with HT—ACOG.
- HRT (estrogen-oral, transdermal, progesterone-oral, and vaginal, intrauterine) or a combined hormonal contraceptive may be offered to women with POI unless contraindicated (for example, in women with hormone-sensitive cancer). Counsel that the baseline population risk of diseases such as breast cancer and cardiovascular disease increases with age and is very low in women aged under 40.
- HRT should not be regarded as being a contraceptive. Hormone treatment with HRT can induce ovulation in POI patients if FSH levels are sup-pressed.
- Ovarian stimulation with drugs such as clomiphene citrate and gonadotropin therapy should not be routinely used as they have no proven benefit. IVF with donor oocytes/embryos has a high success rate, but is not acceptable to all women with POI.

Indian Menopause Society Guidelines 2013, updated 2015: Global Consensus (The International Menopause Society, The North American Menopause Society, The Endocrine Society, The European Menopause and Andropause Society, The Asia Pacific Menopause Federation, The International Osteoporosis Foundation and The Federation of Latin American Menopause Societies), NICE Guidelines, Spanish consensus on premature menopause 2014.

ENDOMETRIOSIS

Suggested approach to menopausal patients with a past and/or symptoms of endometriosis

- Be aware that endometriosis can occur or recur during menopause.
- Be aware of a risk for malignant transformation (although the incidence is likely to be very small).
- Advice the patient to seek medical attention if she experiences endometriosis like symptoms, especially if she is using hormonal replacement therapy (HRT).

- Evaluate the benefit and risks of HRT for the individual patient, considering age, previous disease severity, family history, comorbidities, and BMI.
- Actively engage patient in decision making process and understand our limitation as providers to qualify specific risks.
- If the decision to initiate or continue HRT is made, consider choosing a combined HRT preparation instead of an estrogen-only formulation, taking into consideration the increased risk of breast cancer with combined HRT.
- Consider alternative therapies (e.g. tibolone, aromatase inhibitors, selective estrogen receptor modulators (SERMs) combined with estrogens).
- Consider obtaining tissue for histology if any suspicion of malignancy.

For women with a history of endometriosis who undergo surgical menopause, clinician must balance the benefit of HRT to bone and cardiovascular health against the potential risk of recurrence or malignancy. The decision when to initiate HRT after surgical menopause must be individualized to the patient, considering her age and past medical history.

Gemmell LC, Webster KE, Kirtley S, et al. The management of menopause in women with a history of endometriosis: a systematic review. Hum Reprod Update. 2017;23(4):481–500.

POLYCYSTIC OVARIAN DISEASE

- Polycystic ovarian syndrome (PCOS) is the single most common endocrine metabolic disorder of humans, affecting up to 15% of women. It is characterized by chronic oligo- or anovulation, hyperandrogenism, hyperinsulinemia, dyslipidemia, and metabolic syndrome.
- Within the various studies on PCOS, many different phenotypes of PCOS are identified apart from the classical phenotype (oligo-ovulation, polycystic ovaries and hyperandrogenemia) The transition of women with PCOS into menopause and whether there is a specific phenotype for PCOS after menopause is poorly understood.
- There is evidence that women with PCOS have a larger cohort of primary follicles than age-matched control women before menopause. Serum T levels decrease as women age from the third to fifth decades. Additionally, women with PCOS often develop improved menstrual regularity with age. These factors may all contribute to improvement in reproductive functioning with age before menopause.
- *Diagnosis in perimenopause and menopause:* Menopausal PCOS phenotype is poorly defined. Although there are currently no diagnostic criteria for PCOS in perimenopausal and menopausal women, a presumptive diagnosis of PCOS can be based upon a well-documented long-term history of oligomenorrhea and hyperandrogenism during the productive years. The presence of PCO morphology on ultrasound would provide additional supportive evidence, although this is less likely in a menopausal woman.
- PCOS is a major risk factor for developing impaired glucose tolerance (IGT) and type 2 diabetes (T2D). IGT, and T2D (classic risk indicators of atherosclerosis and CVD) are more prevalent in women with PCOS, even

when weight matched with normal control women. PCOS at any age is characterized by greater odds for an elevated cardiovascular disease (CVD) risk markers. Elevated markers occur without obesity and are magnified with obesity. Dyslipidemia, life-long metabolic dysfunction in women with PCOS exaggerates CVD risk, causing a possible increase in CVD events with age, especially after menopause.

Among non-diabetic postmenopausal women with intact ovaries, atherosclerotic CVD is associated with features of PCOS, such as relative androgen excess and a recalled history of irregular menses.

- Uncertainty exists as to whether PCOS status per se increases cardiovascular mortality. The optimum multifaceted approach to women with PCOS that reduces and prevents CVD has yet to be determined.
- Women with PCOS are three times more likely to develop endometrial carcinoma compared with women without PCOS. Also, present data do not show an increased risk of ovarian or breast cancer in women with PCOS. There is insufficient evidence to evaluate any association of PCOS with vaginal, vulvar or cervical cancer.
- *Management*: Accurate diagnosis of PCOS defined and based on two of the three criteria from the Rotterdam consensus. Blood pressure measurement and fasting blood glucose should be taken. Women with a body mass index greater than 30 or a strong family history of type 2 diabetes should have a glucose tolerance test, particularly if fertility is an issue. All overweight PCOS women should be provided with dietary and lifestyle advice. Amenorrheic or severely oligomenorrheic women with PCOS should have induced withdrawal bleeds at regular intervals to reduce the risk of developing endometrial hyperplasia.

Fauser BC, Tarlatzis BC, Rebar RW, et al. Consensus on women's health: aspects of polycystic ovary syndrome (PCOS): the Amsterdam ESHRE/ASRM-Sponsored 3rd PCOS Consensus Workshop. Fertil Steril. 2012;97:28–38. e25.

Lergo RS, Arslanian SA, Ehrmann DA, et al. A Diagnosis and Treatment of Polycystic Ovary Syndrome: An Endocrine Society Clinical Practice Guideline. J Clin Endocrin Metab. 2013;98(12):4562-92.

Chapter 8

Current Status of Cervical Cancer: Globally and India

Niranjan Chavan

INTRODUCTION

Cervical cancer is the fifth most common cancer in humans, the second most common cancer in women worldwide. It is the most common cause of cancer death in the developing countries. Large majority (around 85%) of the global burden occurs in the less developed regions, where it accounts for almost 12% of all female cancers. Sexually transmitted human papilloma virus (HPV) infection is the most important risk factor for cervical intraepithelial neoplasia and invasive cervical cancer.

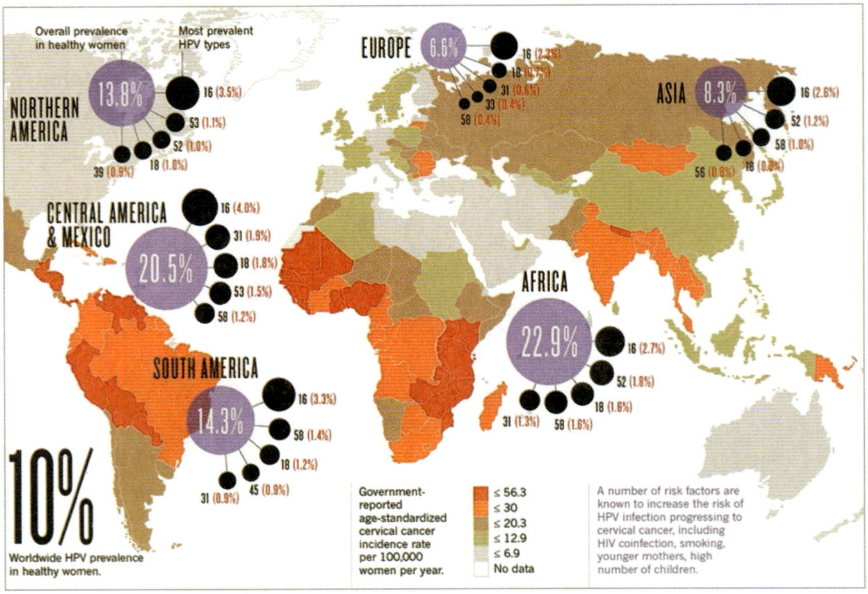

Fig. 1: Worldwide Prevalence of cervical cancer in 2015.

HISTORY AND EVOLUTION

First description of cervical cancer was made by Hippocrates in 400 BC, but it was not until 1834, that cervical cancer was identified as a sexually transmitted disease. In 1928, a Greek cytopathologist Georgios Papanikolaou developed a cervical cytology smear test, today called Pap smear, to detect cancer cells. Harald Zur Hausen and Lutz Gissmann demonstrated the presence of HPV DNA (HPV 16 and HPV 18) in cervical cancer cells in 1985. They were awarded the Noble prize in medicine in 2008 for this revolutionary discovery that paved the foundation for vaccination and prevention against cervical cancer.

GLOBAL BURDEN

Cervical cancer is the second most common cancer in women with an estimated 528,000 new cases in 2016. High-risk regions are defined as region with estimated *age standardized rates* over 30 per 100,000. These include Eastern Africa, Southern and Middle Africa. Cervical cancer remains the most common cancer in women in Eastern and Middle Africa. Lowest age standardized rates, i.e. <7.9 per 100, 000 are seen in Australia/New Zealand and Western Asia.

Even though the prevalence of cervical cancer remains high, but there is a significant decrease in incidence of cervical cancer in most of the ethnic groups according to World Health Organization (WHO) issue on Global health sector strategy on sexually transmitted diseases published in June 2016. There is maximum decrease of 3.9% in Hispanic Women and 1.1% decrease in white women. A substantial decrease by 3.1% per year in mortality due to cervical cancer has been reported among Asian or Pacific Islander women.

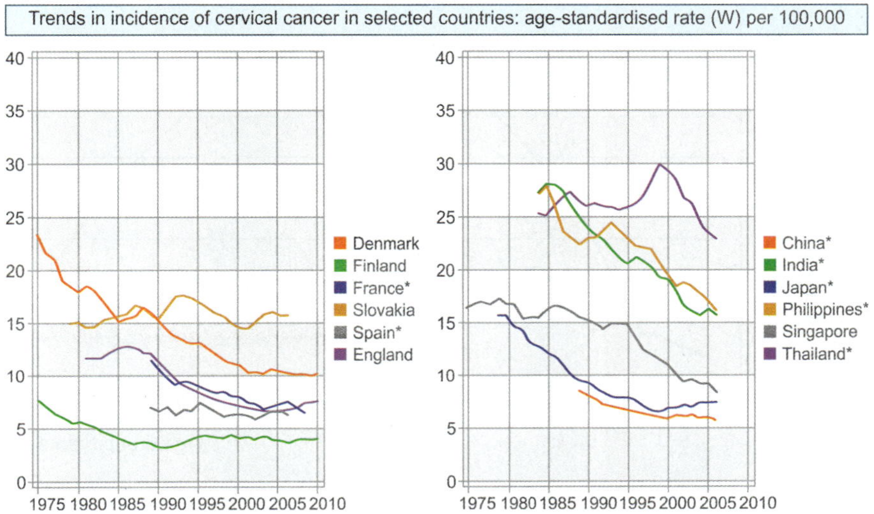

Fig. 2: Data from globocan 2012, international agency for research on cancer, World Health Organization.

INDIAN BURDEN

Cervical cancer is the commonest cancer cause of death among women in India. It is the second most common cancer in women aged 15–44 years. An estimated 122,844 new cases and 67,477 deaths due to cervical cancer occurred in India in 2014, contributing 26% and 27% to the global cervical cancer incidence and mortality respectively. The peak age of incidence of cervical cancer is 55–59 years, and a considerable proportion of women report in the late stages of disease.

India has the highest age standardized incidence of cervical cancer in South Asia at 22, compared to 19.2 in Bangladesh, 13 in Sri Lanka, and 2.8 in Iran. The recent NCRP (National Cancer Registry Program) data show that Aizawl district had the highest levels of cervical cancer at an age-adjusted rate of 24.3, followed by Barshi expanded at 19.5 and Bengaluru at 18.9.

Most factors related to cervical cancer are associated with sexual behavior and it is well-established that Human Papillomavirus (HPV) infections play a critical role in the development of cervical cancer. HPV prevalence among cervical cancer patients in India has varied from 87.8% to 96.67%. The prevalence was higher among high-risk categories such as commercial sex workers at 25%, urban slum in Mumbai at 32.3% and HIV-positive women from 41.7% to 56%. HPV-16 has been found most commonly.

India lacks a nationwide screening program leading to area wise disparities in screening, treatment, and survival. Opportunistic screening in various regions of India varies from 6.9% in Kerala to 0.006% and 0.002% in the western state of Maharashtra and southern state of Tamil Nadu, respectively. Most of the cases present in advanced and late stages, and more than half (63–89%) have locally advanced stage at the time of presentation.

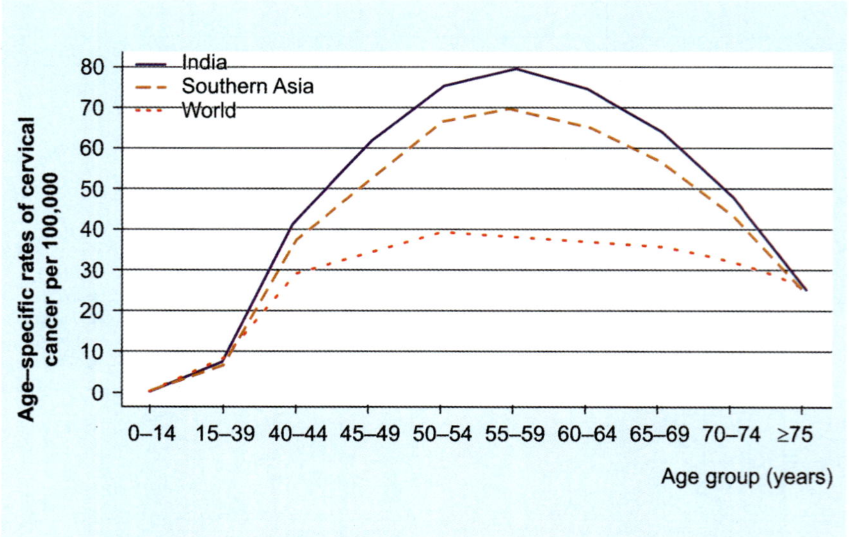

Fig 3: Age-specific incidence rate in India and world. Data recovered from hpvcentre.net/statistics/reports accessed on 10.07.2017.

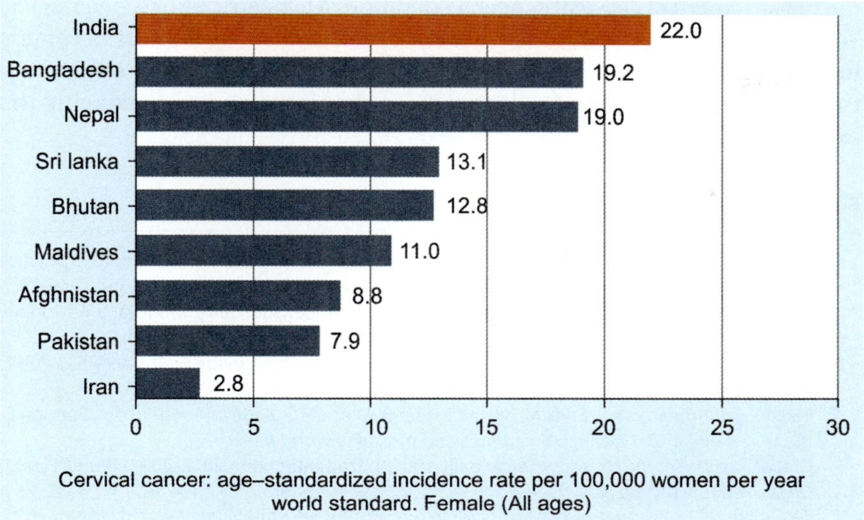

Fig 4: Age-standardized incidence rate of cervical cancer in countries of Southern Asia.

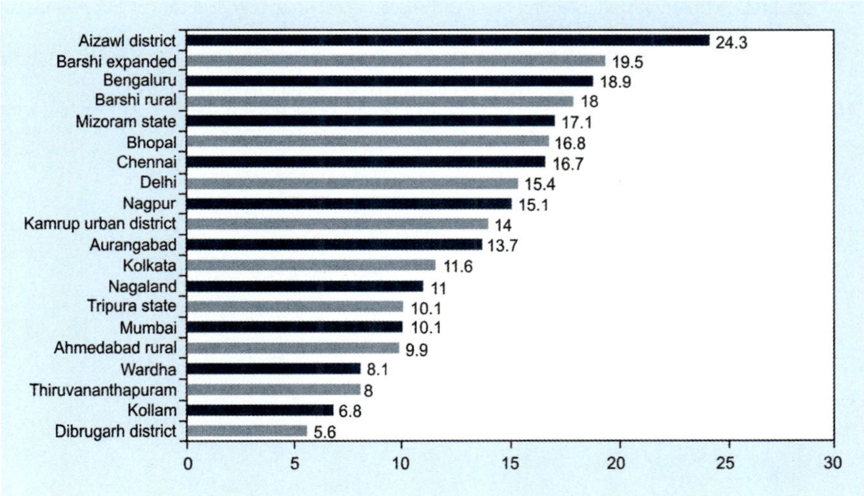

Fig 5: Age standard rates in various regions of India.

WHERE DO WE STAND?

Cervical cancer is the 2nd most common cancer in women worldwide but most common cause of cancer-related death in India. All over the world, including India, there is decreasing trend of cervical cancer. However, where countries like USA are celebrating a substantial decrease in HPV infection owing to their immunization program, in India, women continue to be afflicted by a disease that is potentially preventable and treatable when detected early. Those who are lost to screening or who do not receive screening at all are most susceptible to the development of cervical cancer. Federation of Obstetric and Gynecological Societies of India (FOGSI) has presently started *connecting the dots* 15 centers in India recognized by FOGSI for compiling the data of cervical cancer and training in PAP smear and colposcopy so that it may help in reducing the incidence of cervical cancer.

FURTHER READING

1. Aswathy S, quereshi MA, Kurian B, et al. Cervical cancer screening: current knowledge & practice among women in a rural population of Kerala, India. Indian J. Med Res. 2012;136(2):205-10.
2. Dikshit R, gupta PC, ramasundarahettige C, et al. Cancer mortality in india: a nationally representative survey. Lancet. 2012;379(9828):1807-16.
3. Farooqui HH, Zodpey S. Cervical cancer control in india: taking evidence to action. J Public Health Policy. 2012;33(2):165-72.
4. Ferlay J, soerjomataram I, Ervik M, dikshit R, Eser S, Mathers C, Rebelo M, Parkin dm, Forman D, Bray F. Globocan 2012, cancer incidence and mortality worldwide.
5. Global health sector strategy on sexually transmitted infections 2016-2021, World Health Organization issue; 2016.
6. Globocan 2012: estimated cancer incidence mortality and prevalence worldwide in 2012, international agency for research on cancer, World Health Organization.
7. Http://www.hpvcentre.net/statistics/reports/ind.pdf. Accessed on 18.07.2017.
8. Mckim A, Walter AC, Sheely KM, et al. An economic analysis of cisplatin alone versus cisplatin doublets in the treatment of women with advanced or recurrent cervical cancer. Eur J Gynaecol Oncol. 2016;37(3):353-6.
9. Shastri SS, Mittra I, Mishra GA, et al. Effect of via screening by primary health workers: randomized controlled study in Mumbai, India. J Natl Cancer Inst. 2014;106(3).
10. Sreedevi A, javed R, Dinesh A. Epidemiology of cervical cancer with special focus on India. Int J Womens Health. 2015;7:405-14.

Chapter 9

Conventional and Liquid-based Cytology

Ramani Manoj, Abraham Peedicayil

INTRODUCTION

In the last century, cervical cancer was the most common cause of cancer deaths in women worldwide and continues to be a significant burden in developing countries now.[1] The Papanicolaou (Pap) test and organized screening brought about a remarkable decline in cervical cancer mortality in developed countries.[2] This is the most successful cancer screening test, which has stood the test of time and continues to be a very good method. Discovered and developed by a Greek Anatomist, Georgios Papanicolaou in the US, this is a method of testing for cancer cells in vaginal smears.[3] This later evolved into the more established cervical smears made using Ayre spatula, after the Canadian gynecologist Ernest Ayre who first used wooden spatula to collect samples from the cervix.[4] Eventually, cervical cytology developed into a screening test for cervical neoplasia.

However, the scenario in India is different, as is in most developing countries. In spite of the high burden of cervical cancer, there is no structured screening program. Cytology is not available in many centers and it is mainly opportunistic screening that is being done.

However, it has been established that screening by conventional Papanicolaou (Pap) smears has reduced the mortality by 70%.[5,6] The sensitivity of this screening procedure is 50–60% and reaches 80% at its best[1] and is thus associated with a false-negative rate of 20–50%.[7] In 1996, liquid-based cytology (LBC) method was developed hoping to overcome the disadvantages of the conventional Pap smear. This was expected to have better results such as high sensitivity, sample adequacy, and faster sample preparation. LBC used a different technique and required special collection and preparation set. The LBC method decreased the rate of inadequate smears, and allowed the use of the supernatant for molecular biology testing of viruses such as human papillomavirus (HPV).[8] Some papers have reported no differences between the sensitivity of these two methods, while others have given LBC a higher sensitivity.[9-11] Extra slides prepared from residual LBC sample can upgrade the diagnosis in 14% cases.[12,13]

SAMPLE COLLECTION

A vaginal speculum is used to see the cervix. Sometimes lax vaginal walls or the position of the cervix may make it difficult to actually visualize the cervix. An appropriate speculum or vaginal wall retractors may be needed.

The specimen is collected with an Ayre spatula or cervical brush. There are different types of brushes—broom, bottle, or Christmas tree.

- Turning the wooden Ayre spatula clockwise through two turns (720°)
- Also collect secretions from the posterior fornix (Fig. 1).

The bottle brush can be used to collect an endocervical sample by rotating it within the endocervix. If the broom brush or Christmas tree brush is used, it can simultaneously collect cells from the ectocervix and endocervix, if just the tip is within the endocervical canal.

Conventional Papanicolaou Test

Cells from a vaginal, exocervical or endocervical, specimen are smeared directly onto a glass slide (Figs. 2 and 3).

Fixation should be done immediately. Spray the smear for several seconds at a distance of about 20 cm or drop the slide into an ethanol-ether mixture.

Liquid-based Cytology (ThinPrep or SurePath) Method

Cells from a vaginal, exocervical or endocervical, specimen are collected and transferred into a transport solution medium (Cytyc solution container) by agitating vigorously the collection tool into the solution by rotating it about

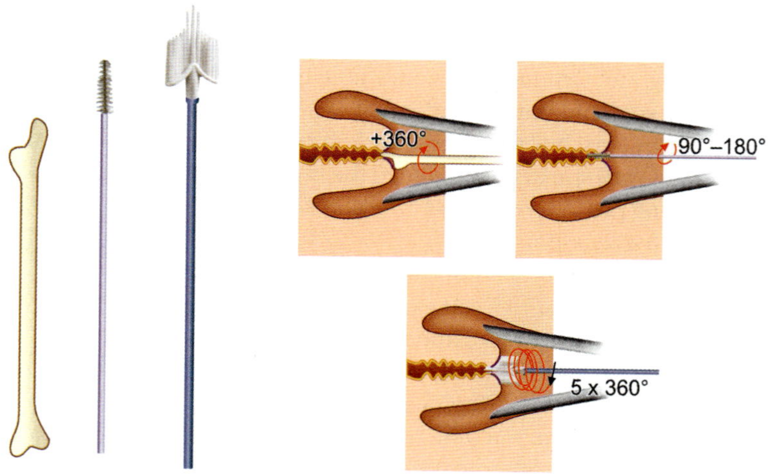

Fig. 1: Sampling devices.

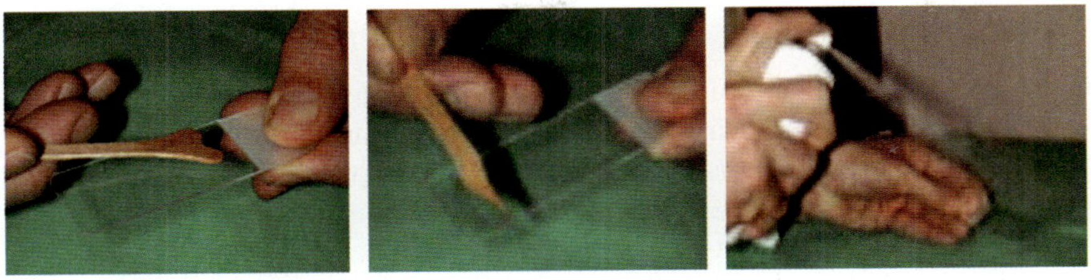

Fig. 2: Preparation of a smear and fixation.

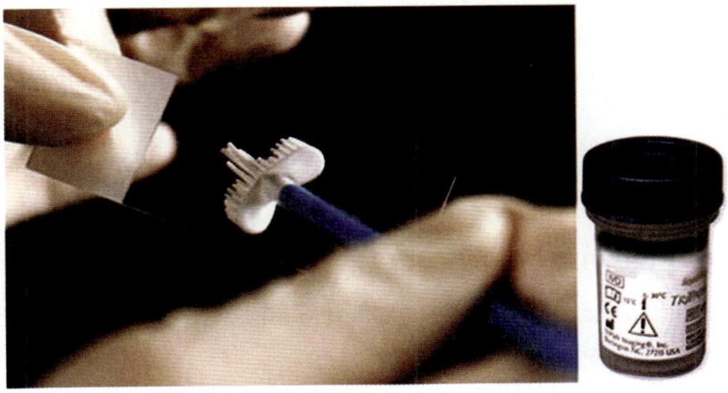

Fig. 3: Preparation of smear with a broom brush.

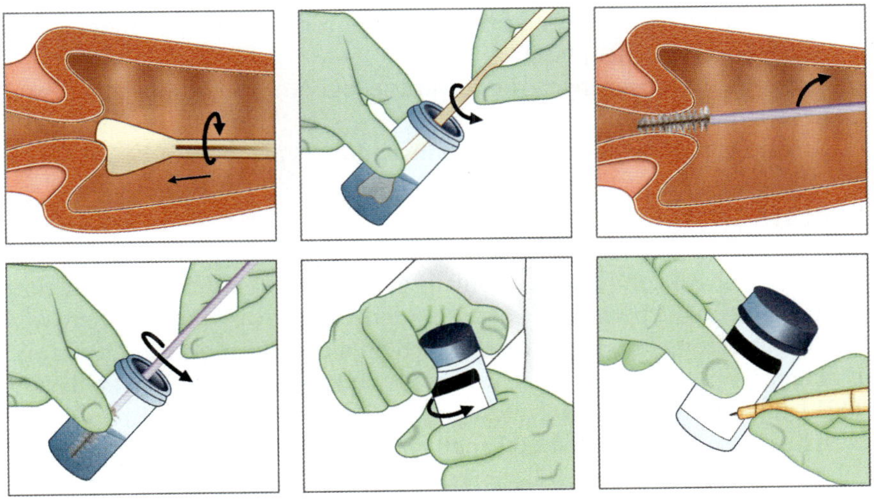

Fig. 4: Sample collection for liquid-based cytology.

10 times. The spatula or brush is discarded. If the brush head is detachable, it may be dropped into the LBC container (Fig. 4).

Label the Specimen

- First and last name
- Age and unique identifying number.

Requisition Form

The requisition form should also have the name, age, and unique identifying number of the woman giving the sample. Indicate the source of the specimen and the last menstrual period of the patient on the pathology requisition.

Send the sample to the laboratory along with the requisition form.

Staining

The Pap stain is a multichromatic stain (not standardized) that imparts different colors to various cell components—nuclei are crisp blue, cells with keratin and glycogen stain yellow, superficial cells are orange to pink, intermediate and parabasal cells are turquoise green while metaplastic cells often stain green and pink simultaneously. Some of the components can interact and precipitate each other, so the shelf life is not long.

Screening Recommendations

- All women who have been sexually active and are above the age of 25 years may be offered the Pap smear.
- The Pap smear may be done every 3 years, if normal.
- Screening may be stopped after age of 65 years, if the previous smears have been normal.
- Those who have had hysterectomy do not require smears unless it was done for cervical neoplasia.
- Those who have been treated for cervical neoplasia or are immunosuppressed need annual screening.
- Screening may be done by either conventional Pap or LBC.

DISCUSSION

In a meta-analysis conducted by Abulafia et al.[14] using 17 articles selected from the literature in the period between 1990 and 2002, it was seen that there was agreement among 89% of the cases based on a classification with five levels of diagnosis [negative, atypical, low-grade squamous intraepithelial lesion (LSIL), high-grade squamous intraepithelial lesion (HSIL), and carcinoma).

It has been reported that LBC method was superior to detect SIL lesions (5.1% vs 3.5%) especially HSIL lesions compared to the conventional Pap smear (1% vs 0.5%). They also reported that detection of the ASCUS and LSIL lesions was lower in LBC than the conventional Pap smear and LBC demonstrated no change in detecting the lesions of squamous cell carcinoma (SCC), adenocarcinoma, and HSIL compared to the conventional Pap smear method.[15]

Setsu Akamatsu and his colleagues in a study published in 2012 concluded that LBC technique has significantly lower percentage of unsatisfactory samples compared to the conventional method (1.4 and 11.5%, $p < 0.01$). It was also noted that repeated screening among women using LBC was better for detection of abnormality compared to conventional method ($p < 0.05$).[16]

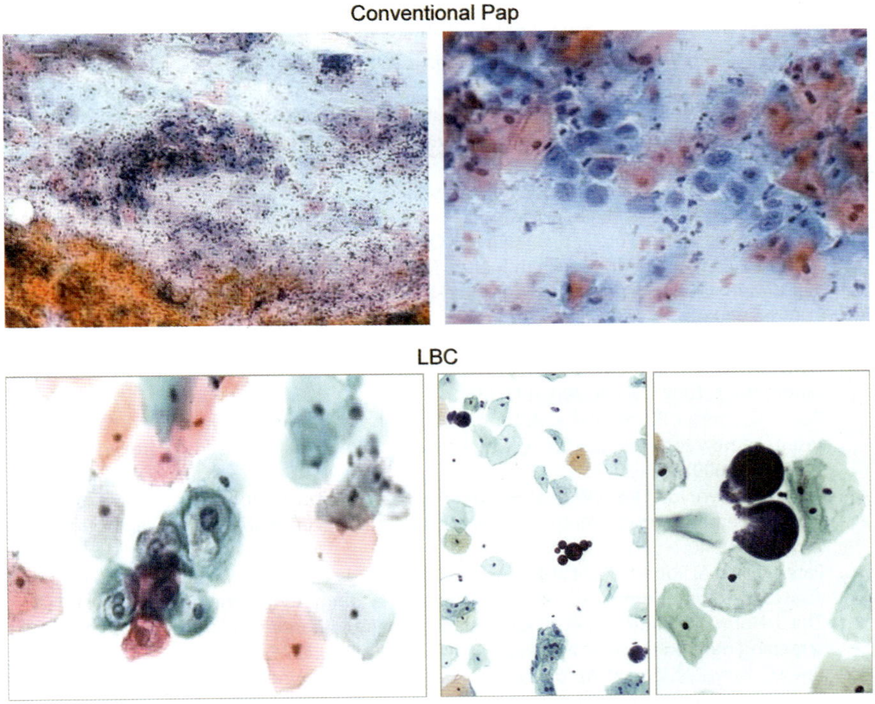

Fig. 5: Comparison of conventional and liquid-based cytology (LBC) smears.

Residual material from LBC can be used for additional slides and ancillary tests such as cell block preparation and molecular studies for HPV and gonorrhea.

Although LBC is more expensive, its widespread introduction to the routine screening will allow the establishment of standards in collection, preparation, and staining of samples that will guarantee an improvement in the quality of testing and diagnostics, as well as reduce possible losses from cytological repetition, and support additional investigation of STIs (sexually transmitted infections).

In a study from Bhutan,[17] the test positivity rate for cytology was 7.5% for a threshold of ASCUS+ and 3.7% for LSIL+. The sensitivity for CIN2+ and CIN3+ was 61% and 74%, respectively. The specificity for CIN2+ and CIN3+ was 94% for both thresholds.

The quality of cytological services will depend—(1) on proper sample collection from the ectocervix and endocervix, (2) proper smear preparation and staining by the cytotechnician, and (3) proper reading and interpretation of the slide with supervision by a cytopathologist. For a successful screening program, there should be adequate coverage, timely follow-up on results, confirmation by biopsy, and appropriate treatment for those with abnormalities. There should be systems for documentation, triage, treatment, and recall of defaulters (Fig. 5).

REFERENCES

1. Parkin DM, Bray FI, Devassa SS. Cancer burden in the year 2000: the global picture. Eur J Cancer. 2001;37:54-66.
2. Siegel R, Naishadham D, Jemal A. Cancer statistics, 2013. CA Cancer J Clin. 2013;63:11-30.
3. Papanicolaou GN, Traut HF. The diagnostic value of vaginal smears in carcinoma of the uterus. Am J Obstet Gynecol. 1941;42:193-206.
4. Ayre JE. Selective cytology smear for diagnosis of cancer. Am J Obstet Gynecol. 1947;53:606-17.
5. Singh E, Seth S, Rani V, et al. Awareness of cervical cancer screening among nursing staff in a tertiary institution of rural India. J Gynecol Oncol. 2012;23:141-6.
6. Mood IN, Dehdashti MR, Eftekhar Z, et al. The specimen adequacy and atypical squamous cell frequency: Conventional versus liquid-based cytology Pap smears. Tehran Univ Med J. 2009;66:900-6.
7. Strander B, Andersson-Ellström A, Milsom I, Rådberg T, et al. Liquid-based cytology versus conventional Papanicolaou smear in an organized screening program: A prospective randomized study. Cancer. 2007;111:285-91.
8. Ronco G, Cuzick J, Pierotti P, et al. Accuracy of liquid-based versus conventional cytology: Overall results of new technologies for cervical cancer screening: Randomised controlled trial. BMJ. 2007;335(7609):28.
9. Treacy A, Reynolds J, Kay EW, et al. Has the ThinPrep method of cervical screening maintained its improvement over conventional smears in terms of specimen adequacy? Diagn Cytopathol. 2009;37:239-40.
10. Patel C, Ullal A, Roberts M, et al. Endometrial carcinoma detected with SurePath liquid-based cervical cytology: Comparison with conventional cytology. Cytopathology. 2009;20:380-7.
11. Zhu J, Norman I, Elfgren K, et al. A comparison of liquid-based cytology and Pap smear as a screening method for cervical cancer. Oncol Rep. 2007;18:157-60.
12. Chen C, Yang Z, Li Z, et al. Accuracy of several cervical screening strategies for early detection of cervical cancer: A meta-analysis. Int J Gynecol Cancer. 2012;22:908-21.
13. Grapsa D, Ioakim-Liossi A, Stergiou E, et al. Additional slides from residual ThinPrep Pap tests: Of potential diagnostic benefit in equivocal cases? Diagn Cytopathol. 2012;40:856-60.
14. Abulafia O, Pezzullo JC, Sherer DM. Performance of ThinPrep liquid-based cervical cytology in comparison with conventionally prepared Papanicolaou smears: a quantitative survey. Gynecol Oncol. 2003;90:137-44.
15. Mills SE, Carter D, Gresson JK, et al. Sternberg's diagnostic Surgical pathology, 4th edition. Philadelphia; Lippincott Williams and Wilkins: 2004. pp 2377-8.
16. Akamatsua S, Kodamac S, Himejia Y, et al. Comparison of Liquid-based Cytology with Conventional Cytology in Cervical Cancer Screening. Acta Cytologica. 2012;56:370-4.
17. Tshomo U, Franceschi S, Tshokey T, et al. Evaluation of cytology versus human papillomavirus-based cervical cancer screening algorithms in Bhutan. Oncotarget. 2017;8:72438-46.

APPENDIX

The interpretation categories of the 2014 Bethesda system for reporting cervical cytology are as follows:

I. NEGATIVE FOR INTRAEPITHELIAL LESION OR MALIGNANCY

- **Non-neoplastic findings:**
  - Non-neoplastic cellular variations:
    - ◊ Squamous metaplasia
    - ◊ Keratotic changes
    - ◊ Tubal metaplasia
    - ◊ Atrophy
    - ◊ Pregnancy-associated changes
  - Reactive cellular changes associated with:
    - ◊ Inflammation
    - ◊ Radiation
    - ◊ Intrauterine contraceptive device
  - Glandular cells status posthysterectomy.
- **Organisms:**
  - *Trichomonas vaginalis*
  - *Candida species*
  - Bacterial vaginosis
  - *Actinomyces*
  - Herpes simplex virus
  - Cytomegalovirus.

II. OTHER

Endometrial cells (in a woman ≥45 years of age).

III. EPITHELIAL CELL ABNORMALITIES

- **Squamous cell:**
  - Atypical squamous cells:
    - ◊ of undetermined significance (ASC-US)
    - ◊ cannot exclude HSIL (ASC-H)
  - Low-grade squamous intraepithelial lesion (LSIL)
  - High-grade squamous intraepithelial lesion (HSIL)
    - ◊ with features suspicious for invasion
  - Squamous cell carcinoma.
- **Glandular cell:**
  - Atypical:
    - ◊ Endocervical cells
    - ◊ Endometrial cells
    - ◊ Glandular cells
  - Atypical:
    - ◊ Endocervical cells, favor neoplastic
    - ◊ Glandular cells, favor neoplastic
  - Endocervical adenocarcinoma in situ

- Adenocarcinoma:
  - ◊ Endocervical
  - ◊ Endometrial
  - ◊ Extrauterine
  - ◊ Not otherwise specified.

IV. OTHER MALIGNANT NEOPLASMS

Adequacy is also commented upon, in the report: satisfactory/unsatisfactory (the latter with reasons such as rejected, not processed, etc.)

Many epithelial reports too have comments following them, to specify either the abnormality or infection, as is the case.

Chapter 10

Swede Score and IFCPC 2011 Nomenclature in Interpretation of Colposcopy Findings

Dipanwita Banerjee, Manisha Vernekar, Ranajit Mandal

BACKGROUND

Introduction of noncytological screening tests like visual inspection with 3–5% acetic acid, human papillomavirus deoxyribonucleic acid (DNA) test has made the role of colposcopy more important in cervical cancer screening. Colposcopy plays a central role in the management of patients with abnormal screening tests. To improve the examination findings, various colposcopic indexes like Reid index, Swede Score have been introduced to interpret colposcopic findings followed by with/without biopsy as the gold standard. In all scoring systems invented till date, cutoff scores are set for different cervical lesion grades, which greatly simplify the evaluations and make them easy to learn. However, there are discrepancies when correlation studies are being done between various colposcopic scoring systems with histology findings.[1] To validate the interpretations, repeated efforts have been made to unify the colposcopic nomenclature of the findings which will improve the diagnostic accuracy of colposcopy.

IMPORTANCE OF SWEDE SCORE

The Reid's colposcopy index (RCI), most well-known scoring system, was first reported by Reid and Scalzi in 1985[2] and was shown to have good consistency of strength kappa as 0.55–0.74 with histopathology in several reports.[3-5] However, in the results of the ASCUS LSIL Triage Study (ALTS) showed poor agreement between the modified RCI and histopathology and poor reproducibility amongst the colposcopists.[6-8]

Recognizing the correlation of size of the lesion with probability of harboring high-grade disease, a new scoring system, the Swede score, has been proposed by Strander et al. in 2005.[9] In addition to the various parameters of RCI, Swede score also incorporates lesion size as a variable. Table 1 describes the variables for reporting the Swede score findings. The total score ranges between 0 to 10, assigning each parameter a score between 0 to 2. A score of more than equal to 5 is reported to identify all high-grade squamous intraepithelial lesions (HSIL). A score less than 5 is not of much interest as normal metaplastic changes may also turn acetowhite on application of 3–5% acetic acid. Therefore biopsy can be avoided in these cases. A score between 5–7 is an indication for biopsy due to likelihood of low-grade squamous intraepithelial lesion (LSIL). A score more than equal to 8 is suggestive of high-grade lesions including early invasive disease hence can directly go for excision treatment, which is both diagnostic and therapeutic in the management of cervical precancers. Over last decade Swede Score has proved its validity in management of cervical precancers.[10-12]

Evidence suggests higher the cutoff, the specificity increases with loss in sensitivity (sensitivity 95% vs. specificity <40%), whereas lowering the cutoff to 6 improves the sensitivity and also with high-negative predictive value at the expense of specificity (sensitivity 65% vs. specificity 82%).[9,11] In low resource settings, where maximum utilization of resources and coverage of maximum number of high-risk women is required, performing treatment as a "see and treat" approach at this cutoff is feasible. By treating the women who are truly at risk of developing cervical cancer, single visit approach with a specific cutoff on colposcopy findings is appropriate and thus reduces the burden of failure to receive treatment. There are studies which showed usefulness of Swede score in evaluating abnormal cytology in pregnant women and may even reduce the need for diagnostic biopsies.

INTERNATIONAL FEDERATION FOR CERVICAL PATHOLOGY AND COLPOSCOPY COLPOSCOPIC TERMINOLOGY

In 2011, the International Federation for Cervical Pathology and Colposcopy (IFCPC) presented the new international colposcopic terminology or

Table 1: Swede score for interpretation of colposcopy findings.

	Score		
	0	*1*	*2*
Uptake of acetic acid	0 or transparent	Shady and milky	Distinct and stearin like
Margins and Surface	0 or diffuse	Sharp, but irregular, jagged, and "geographical" satellites	Sharp and even, difference in surface level such as "cutting"
Vessels	Fine and regular	Absent	Coarse or atypical
Lesion size	<5 mm	5–15 mm or spanning 2 quadrants	>15 mm or spanning 3–4 quadrants or endocervically undefined
Iodine staining	Brown	Faintly or patchy yellow	Distinct yellow

classification system at the 14th World Congress in Rio de Janeiro. The proposed classification was based on the versions developed in 1975, 1990, and 2002.[13,14] The main objective of this classification is to make colposcopy finding more reproducible and easy to understand and document the exact finding which is being seen. The details of the Classification are given in Table 2.

The notable points of the proposed nomenclature are:

1. The first step is to assess whether the colposcopy is representative. General assessment for colposcopy examination by three variables, including the

Table 2: IFCPC 2011 colposcopy terminology classification.

General assessment		❑ Adequate or inadequate (reason) ❑ *SCJ visible:* Completely visible or partially visible or not visible ❑ *Transformation zone:* 1/2/3	
Normal colposcopic findings		*Original squamous epithelium:* ❑ Mature ❑ Trophic *Columnar epithelium:* ❑ Ectopy *Metaplastic squamous epithelium:* ❑ Nabothian cysts ❑ Crypt openings ❑ Deciduosis in pregnancy	
Abnormal colposcopic findings	*General principles*	*Location of the lesion: Inside TZ or Outside TZ* ❑ Clock position (please mark below) ❑ Number of quadrants involved:1/2/3/4 ❑ *Size of lesion:* <25%/25–50%/50–75%/>75%	
	Grade 1 (Minor)	❑ Thin AW epithelium ❑ Irregular and geographic border	❑ Fine mosaic ❑ Fine punctuation
	Grade 2 (Major)	❑ Dense AW epithelium ❑ Rapid appearance of acetowhitening ❑ Cuffed crypt openings	❑ Coarse mosaic ❑ Coarse punctuation ❑ Sharp border ❑ Inner border sign ❑ Ridge sign
	Nonspecific	❑ Leukoplakia ❑ Erosion ❑ *Lugol's staining (Schiller's test):* Stained or nonstained	
Suspicious for invasion		❑ Atypical vessels ❑ *Additional signs:* Fragile vessels, irregular surface, exophytic lesion, necrosis, ulceration (necrotic), and tumor or gross neoplasm	
Miscellaneous finding		❑ CTZ ❑ Condyloma ❑ Polyp/Inflammation	❑ Stenosis ❑ Congenital anomaly ❑ Post-treatment ❑ Endometriosis

(SCJ: squamocolumnar junction; TZ: transformation zone; AW: Acetowhite; CTZ: congenital transformation zone)

importance of visibility of squamocolumnar junction, three transformation zones (TZ) types, i.e. type 1, 2 and 3 TZ. Most commonly used terms "satisfactory" and "unsatisfactory" colposcopy have been replaced by "adequate" and "inadequate" colposcopy examinations which include reason for inadequacy for future reference.
2. The approach to colposcopy examination is more simple following the steps of colposcopy and description of the findings starts from whether or not the findings are normal.
3. Introduction of two new signs, inner border sign and ridge sign under the heading of Grade II or major grade lesion are proved to have good predictive accuracy, while iodine negativity postulates an inferior performance.
4. Introduced for the first time the types of excision,[13] which represent the latest understanding globally on precancerous lesions of the lower genital tract in women.

This nomenclature emphasizes the importance of various normal or abnormal colposcopic findings more than other colposcopic indexes. Although this IFCPC document presents descriptive terminology rather than a colposcopic index, the classification indicates which patterns of colposcopic findings should be suspected as a benign, low-grade lesions, high-grade lesions and invasive cancer in much elaborate way possible.

CONCLUSION

Introduction of these two relatively new colposcopic classification systems have brought a new approach in dealing of cervix lesions in much simplistic and practical way. Though with HSIL as the cutoff, performance of the comprehensive indexes are better as those with LSIL as the cutoff.[15,16] Both IFCPC colposcopy terminology and Swede score can be used to categorize the cervical abnormalities considering all the variables and possible findings seen while performing colposcopy.

REFERENCES

1. Baum ME, Rader JS, Gibb RK, et al. Colposcopic accuracy of obstetrics and gynecology residents. Gynecol Oncol. 2006;103(3):966-70.
2. Li Y, Duan X, Sui L, et al. Closer to a Uniform Language in Colposcopy: Study on the Potential Application of 2011 International Federation for Cervical Pathology and Colposcopy Terminology in Clinical Practice. BioMed Res Int. 2017;2017:8984516.
3. Mousavi AS, Fakour F, Gilani MM, et al. A prospective study to evaluate the correlation between reid colposcopic index impression and biopsy histology. J Low Genit Tract Dis. 2017;11(3):147-50.
4. Shojaei H, Yarandi F, Ghozati L, et al. Acceptable predictive accuracy of histopathology results by colposcopy done by Gynecology residents using Reid index. Arch Gynecol Obstet. 2013;287(2):345-9.
5. Durdi GS, Sherigar BY, Dalal AM, et al. Correlation of colposcopy using reid colposcopic index with histopathology- a prospective study. J Turk Ger Gynecol Assoc. 2009;10(4):205-7.
6. Ferris DG, Litaker MS, ALTS Group. Prediction of cervical histologic results using an abbreviated Reid Colposcopic Index during ALTS. Am J Obstet Gynecol. 2006;194(3):704-10.

7. Massad LS, Jeronimo J, Schiffman M. Interobserver agreement in the assessment of components of colposcopic grading." Obstet Gynecol. 2008;111(6):1279-84.
8. Massad LS, Jeronimo J, Katki HA, et al. "The accuracy of colposcopic grading for detection of high-grade cervical intraepithelial neoplasia," J Low Genit Tract Dis. 2009;13(3):137-44.
9. Strander B, Ellström-Andersson A, Franzén S, et al. The performance of a new scoring system for colposcopy in detecting high-grade dysplasia in the uterine cervix. Acta Obstet Gynecol Scand. 2005;84(10):1013-7.
10. Kärrberg C, Ryd W, Strander B, et al. Histological diagnosis and evaluation of the swede score colposcopic system in a large cohort of pregnant women with atypical cervical cytology or cervical malignancy signs. Acta Obstet Gynecol Scand. 2012;91(8):952-8.
11. Nessa A, Wistrand C, Begum SA, et al. Evaluation of stationary colposcope and the Gynocular®, by the swede score systematic colposcopic system in VIA positive women: A crossover randomized trial. Int J Gynecol Cancer. 2014;24(2):339-45.
12. Basu P, Banerjee D, Mittal S, et al. Evaluation of a compact, rechargeable, magnifying device to triage VIA and HPV positive women in a cervical cancer screening program in rural India. Cancer Causes Control. 2016;27(10):1253-9.
13. Stafl A. New nomenclature for colposcopy. Report of the committee on terminology. Obstet Gynecol. 1976;48(1):123-4.
14. Stafl A, Wilbanks GD. An international terminology of colposcopy: report of the nomenclature committee of the international federation of cervical pathology and colposcopy. Obstet Gynecol. 1991;77(2):313-4.
15. Walker P, Dexeus S, De Palo G, et al. International terminology of colposcopy: an updated report from the international federation for cervical pathology and colposcopy. Obstet Gynecol. 2003;101(1):175-7.
16. Apgar BS, Kaufman AJ, Bettcher C, et al. Gynecologic procedures: colposcopy, treatments for cervical intraepithelial neoplasia and endometrial assessment. Am Fam Physician. 2013;87(12):836-43.

Chapter 11

Basics of Colposcopy in Detection of Precancerous Lesions

Priya Ganesh Kumar

INTRODUCTION

The history of colposcopy began in March 1924. Due to the practical difficulty in adjusting the focal length, colposcopic examination was almost impossible. This challenge was addressed very efficiently by Hinselmann, a German Clinician and developed the Science of Colposcopy. With scientific additions made to it to improvise the technique the "ART of Colposcopy" was born.

Hence, *Hinselmann* is rightly called the *"Father of Colposcopy".*

Colposcopy allows the service provider to have a magnified view of the cervix and its vasculature.

TERMINOLOGIES

Squamous Epithelium

The original squamous epithelium is pinkish in color. It is multilayered with basal, parabasal, intermediate and superficial cells layer. The superficial layers contain glycogen. They are called stratified squamous epithelium. They turn mahogany brown on application of Lugol's iodine. In case of menopausal age group, the upper layer of superficial layers disappears with only basal, parabasal, and intermediate. This epithelium appears lusterless and do not turn brown.

Columnar Epithelium

This is single layer thrown into folds called crypts. The blocking of the crypt openings give rise to nabothian follicles.

The usual blood vessel pattern found in the cervix is reticular pattern, branching tree like pattern, smooth tapering pattern. In case of lesions, we find bizarre-shaped blood vessel pattern in the shape of broken thread, comma, waste thread, etc.

Squamocolumnar Junction

Squamocolumnar junction (SCJ) is the junction between squamous epithelium and columnar epithelium.

Old SCJ is noted by arbitrary line joining the distal crypt openings.

New SCJ is junction between metaplastic squamous epithelium and columnar epithelium.

Transformation Zone

Transformation zone (TZ) is the zone between old SCJ and new SCJ. They are of three types:

- *Type 1 TZ:* When the new SCJ is completely visible.
- *Type 2 TZ:* The new SCJ is on the cervical os, visible with certain maneuvering.
- *Type 3 TZ:* The new SCJ is completely withdrawn into the cervical canal and is visible on endocervical speculum examination.

Metaplasia

It is the transformation of one epithelium into another.

Squamous Metaplasia

Transformation of columnar epithelium to squamous epithelium. In case of immature squamous metaplasia, the epithelium lacks stratification, i.e. superficial layers with glycogen. Over due course, the immature squamous epithelium develops the superficial layers and hence becomes mature squamous metaplasia. There is no practical difference in mature squamous metaplastic epithelium and original squamous epithelium.

As a Colposcopist one should be proficient to appreciate the *Mosaics and Punctuation* on the lesion. These are related to the caliber of the stromal capillary blood vessels present in the stromal papillae which provides nourishment to the dividing cells. The dividing cells need more nutrients, which are provided by the dilated blood vessels which appears like punctuation spots on head on view during colposcopy examination. So the fine and coarse punctuations represent the less dividing and more dividing cells respectively. Mosaics represent the dividing cells in the Rete pegs. The precancerous cells are very actively dividing cells within the Rete pegs. The mosaic patterns are tiled pavered block like pattern developing due to the accumulated cells in the Rete pegs. The 3D view of the blood vessels surrounding the Rete pegs from the head on view during the colposcopy examination is responsible for the mosaic pattern. Fine and coarse mosaicism depicts the lesion severity.

Getting all the findings on one area of geographical defined pattern arising from SCJ within the TZ, i.e. abnormal blood vessels, acetowhiteness, Lugol's negative is mandatory to understand the cervical intraepithelial neoplasia (CIN) lesion and grading the lesion as per Swede scoring.

Colposcopy with guided biopsy is the gold standard to detect CIN lesions.

COLPOSCOPY EXAMINATION

The steps to be followed in colposcopy examination are discussed here.

1. *Cleaning with normal saline:* On cleaning with normal saline, the cervical discharge is removed. We can take cervical scrape for cytology, HPV before cleaning with normal saline (Fig. 1).
    - I. *Columnar epithelium:* This appears as grape like reddish epithelium. Since columnar epithelium are single layered the underlying stromal blood vessels are clearly visible as reddish color.
    - II. *Islands of columnar epithelium:* These are sometimes visible as small patch of columnar epithelium, identified by its color and grape-like texture.
    - III. *Crypt opening:* To identify the original SCJ, we have to look out for distal crypt opening which appears as depression. Arbitrarily joining the distal crypts gives us an idea of old/original SCJ prior to occurrence of metaplasia.
    - IV. *New SCJ:* Appears as sharp demarcation boundary between the columnar and squamous epithelium. The new SCJ is more highlighted as white line on application of acetic acid.
    - V. *TZ:* Transformation zone between the original arbitrary SCJ and new SCJ. This signifies the metaplastic epithelium
    - VI. *Original Squamous epithelium:* Squamous epithelium being multilayered appears pinkish red. The original squamous epithelium is usually located distal to the distal crypt openings.
    - VII. Immature metaplasia: Appears thin translucent whitish highlighted more on application of 5% acetic acid.
    - VIII. Mature metaplasia appears more pinkish white.
    - IX. *Reticular blood vessel pattern:* The stromal blood vessels appears as reticular mesh pattern seen usually on the squamous epithelium (near SCJ).

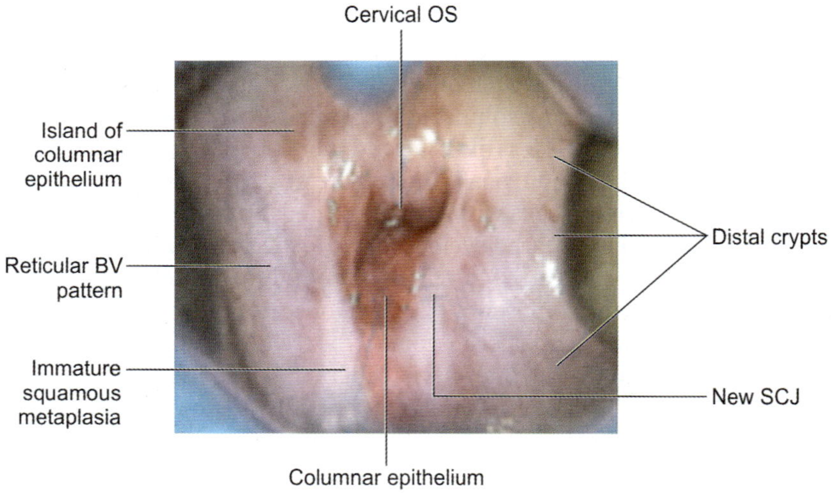

Fig. 1: Cervix after cleaning with normal saline.

2. *Blue green filter:* The blood vessel pattern gets perfectly highlighted with blue green filter.
   Usually, a typical blood vessel pattern is noted on the cervix, the knowledge of which is important to identify the abnormal vascular pattern (Figs. 2A to D). These are the stromal blood vessels forming a pattern. They are highlighted in blue green filter (Fig. 3). The two common types of vascular pattern noted are—reticular and hairpin-shaped pattern. Regular tree branching pattern is seen on the nabothian follicles. Parallel vascular pattern is seen on the healing tissues. Infection with trichomoniasis, the hairpin-shaped vessels assumes staghorn like shapes.
   The vessel patterns in pathological conditions are depicted in Figures 3 and 4.
3. *Application of 5% Acetic Acid:* Principle—acetic acid coagulates the intracellular proteins thus obscuring the passage of light, thus turning acetowhite (Fig. 5).
   Columnar epithelium, mature squamous metaplasia and original squamous epithelium do not turn since there is very less intracellular proteins.
   In case of immature squamous metaplasia, the cells are dividing cells with high nucleocytoplasmic ratio. On application of 5% acetic acid , immature

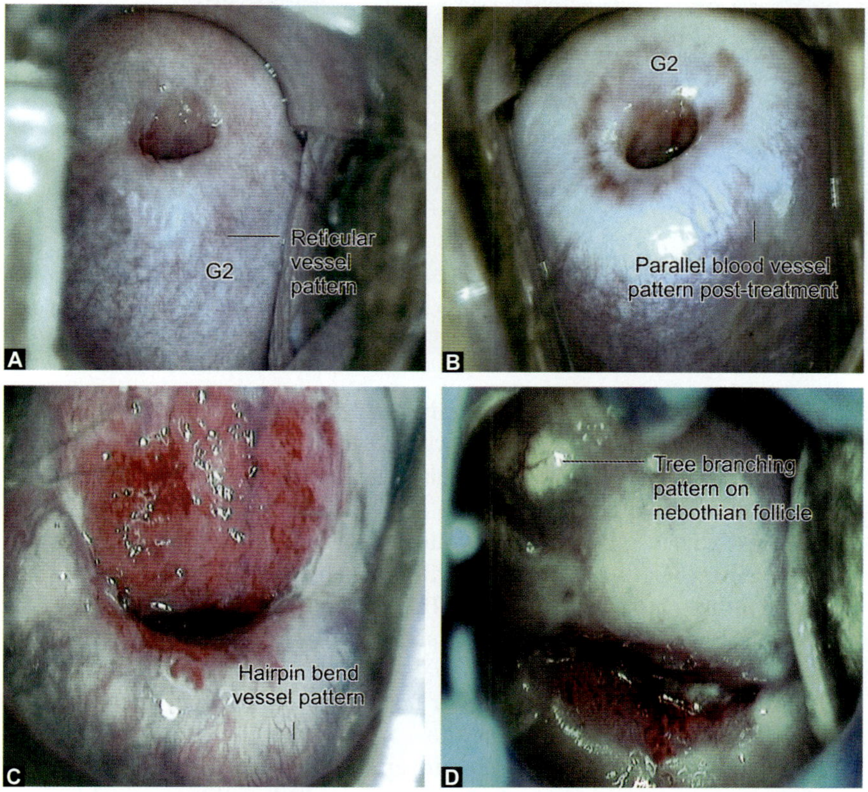

Figs. 2A to D: (A) Reticular vessel pattern. (B) Parallel blood vessel pattern post treatment. (C) Hairpin bend vessel pattern. (D) Tree branching pattern on nabothian follicle.

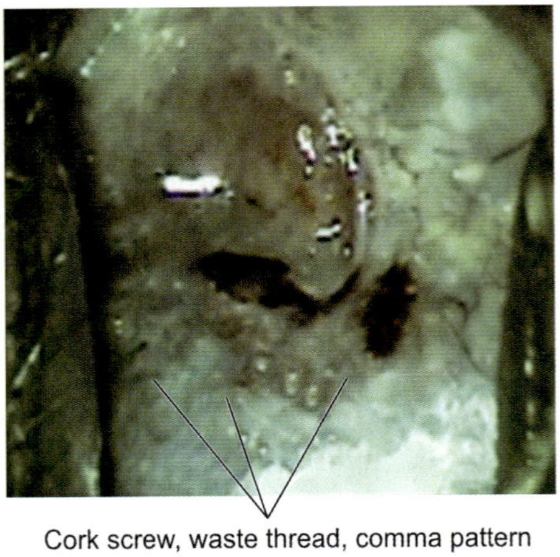

Fig. 3: Low-grade squamous cell intraepithelial lesions (LSIL) irregular blood vessel pattern on blue-green filter of cervix.

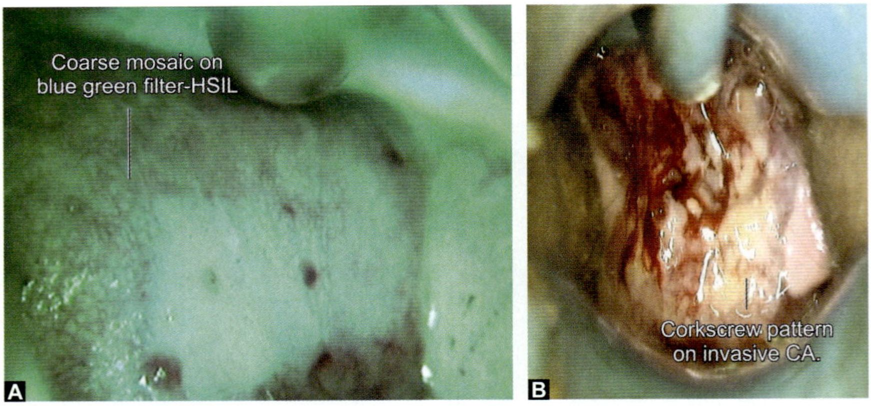

Figs. 4A and B: Vessel patterns in pathological conditions of cervix. (A) Coarse mosaic on blue-green filter (high-grade squamous cell intraepithelial lesions). (B) Corkscrew pattern on invasive carcinoma.

metaplastic tissue turns acetowhite, which is thin, transparent, shiny, without any geographical pattern with finger like or feathery margins. They can arise focally anywhere on the columnar epithelium. The acetowhiteness disappears very quickly.

In case of CIN lesions, the acetowhite lesions have set geographical pattern arising from SCJ within the TZ distributed centrifugally. Low-grade lesions have feathery but distinct margin. They are milky white translucent. High-grade lesions have distinct margin, sometimes elevated rolled out margins, with distinct oyster egg white or chalky white (Figs. 6A and B). Low-grade lesions appear late and disappear fast, whereas the high-grade lesions appear instantly and disappear late.

Sometimes, the columnar epithelium appears white due to the metaplastic changes occurring on them. SCJ appears as a distinct thin acetowhite line.

VIA Positive cases (acetowhite conditions which can be physiological):

- New SCJ
- Squamous metaplasia
- Columnar epithelium covered with immature squamous metaplasia
- Satellite lesions, which is acetowhite within or outside the TZ zone
- Congenital TZ
- Hyperkeratic patches.

VIA positive lesions (acetowhite in pathological conditions):
- LSIL
- HSIL
- Invasive CA
- Microcondylomatous lesion.

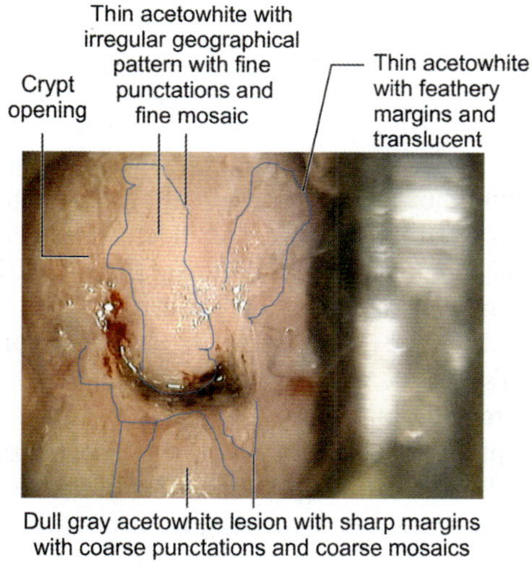

Fig. 5: CIN 1 lesions on upper lip with CIN 2 lesions on lower lip.

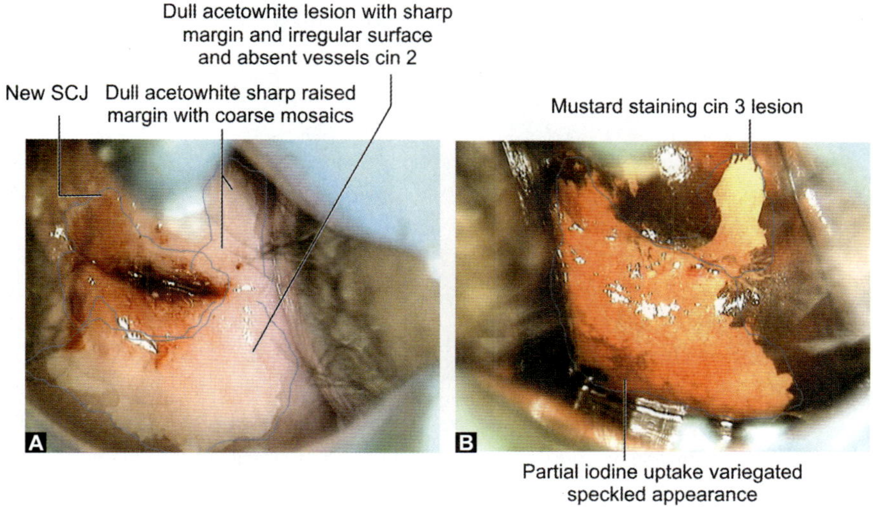

Figs. 6A and B: (A) High-grade CIN 2 lesions at the lower lip and CIN 3 at the upper lip. (B) High-grade lesions with CIN 3 at the upper lip and CIN 2 at the lower lip.

4. *Lugol's Application:* Principle—stratified squamous epithelium has glycogen in their superficial cells. On application of Lugol's iodine, these cells take up iodine and turn Mahogany brown or dark brown. The cells which do not contain glycogen do not turn brown, they remain unstained or variegated patchy appearance.

Physiological conditions where Lugol's is taken up and turns Mahogany brown (VILI negative)—original squamous epithelium, mature squamous metaplasias.

Physiological conditions where Lugol is not taken up-(VILI positive)—columnar epithelium, Immature squamous epithelium, nabothian follicle, menopausal epithelium.

Pathological Conditions not taking up Lugol's Iodine (VILI Positive)

CIN lesions: Due to the lack of superficial stratified cells in the dividing cells of CIN lesions which are usually basal, parabasal or intermediate cells, these lesions do not stain brown. Depending on the severity of the CIN lesions, they either remain unstained or take up partial variegated Lugol's stains, higher-grade lesions such as microinvasive CA stain as mustard yellow (Figs. 7 to 10).

Trichomonial infections cause denudation of the superficial cells which do not get stained giving rise to *leopard* skin pattern.

Satellite lesions which are not arising from SCJ within or away from TZ do not stain with Lugol's and are VILI positive.

Thus to sum up the terminology:

- *VILI Negative:* Uptake of Lugol's iodine to turn into mahogany brown color.
- *VILI Positive:* There is no Lugol's iodine uptake hence they remain unstained or turn yellow, seen in physiological or pathological conditions.

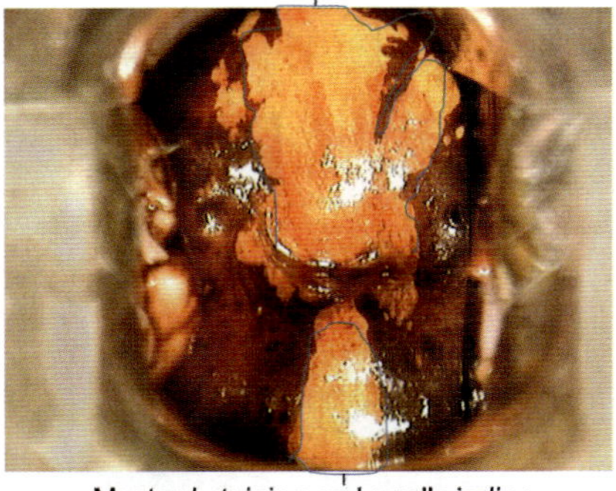

Fig. 7: Mustard staining on Lugol's iodine application iodine negative—high-grade lesion.

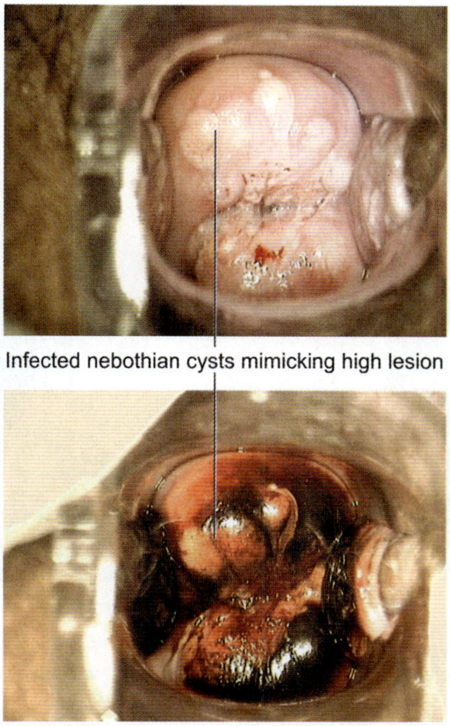

Fig. 8: Nabothian cysts.

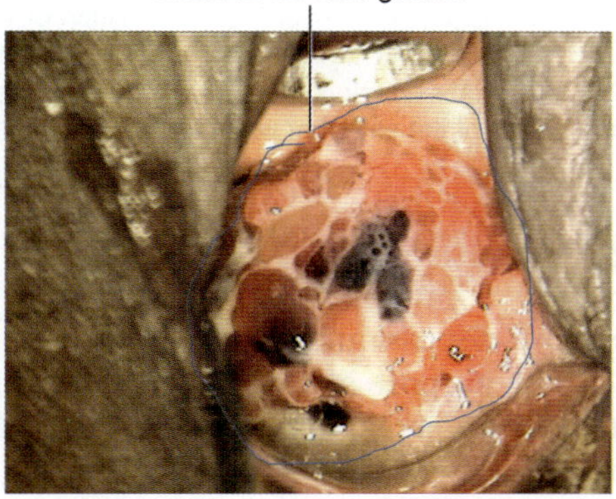

Fig. 9: Necrotic cancer growth flushed with the cervix.

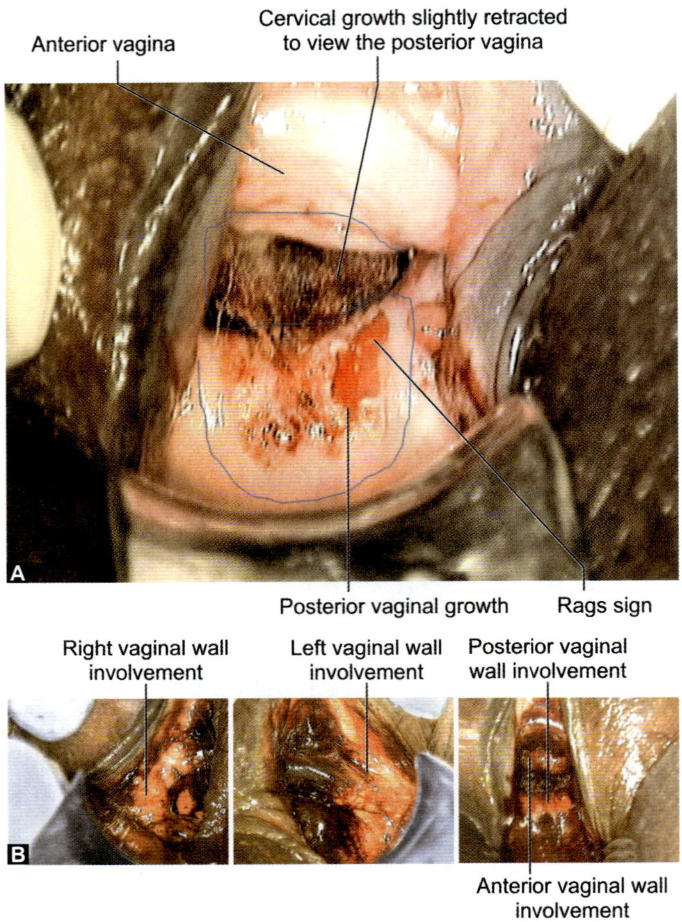

Figs. 10A and B: (A) Vaginal extension of invasive squamous cell cancer (SCC). (B) Demarcation of the extent of vaginal involvement in SCC.

CONCLUSION

It is clear from the above discussion that *colposcopy* is an art and science to identify the lesion for the purpose of biopsy. Once the lesion is identified, it has to be represented by Cartier diagram. Preventive Oncology is a team work of Clinician, Colposcopist, Cytopathologist.

Chapter 12

Management of Cervical Intraepithelial Neoplasia

Geeta Gupta

INTRODUCTION

Cervical intraepithelial neoplasia (CIN) is a histopathological description of premalignant lesion of cervix, in which a part or the full thickness of stratified squamous epithelium is replaced by cells showing varying degrees of dysplasia, however basement membrane is intact. In 1976, Richart proposed the term cervical intraepithelial neoplasia, which combined the categories of severe dysplasia and carcinoma in situ into term CIN 3.

It is estimated that approximately 1–2% of women have CIN2+ each year (Fig. 1). This rate is reported to be higher in women of HIV-positive status,

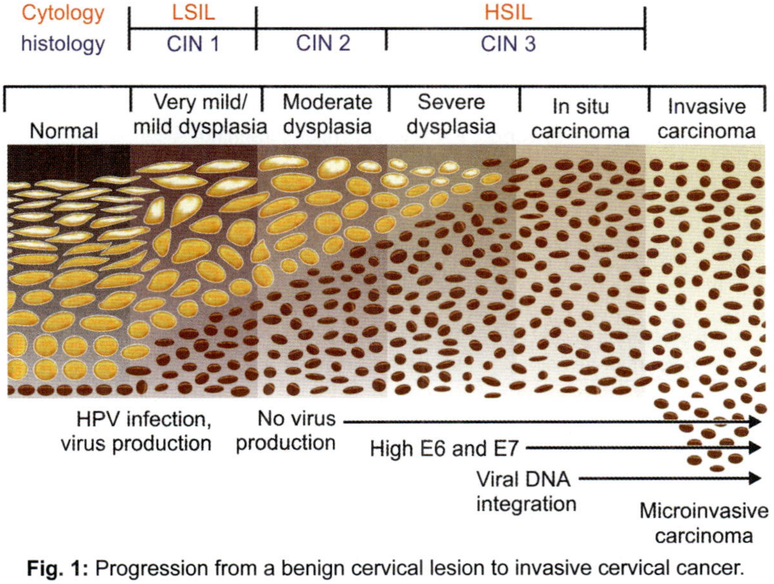

Fig. 1: Progression from a benign cervical lesion to invasive cervical cancer.

(CIN: cervical intraepithelial neoplasia; HSIL: high-grade squamous intraepithelial lesion; LSIL: low-grade squamous intraepithelial lesion)

at 10%. More than 90% of CIN is attributed to human papilloma virus (HPV) infection.

CERVICAL CANCER SCREENING

World Health Organization (WHO) recommends cervical cancer screening should not start before 30 years of age, as cervical cancer is rare and transient high-risk HPV infection is very common before 30 (Table 1). Thus cervical cancer screening is recommended for every woman between ages of 30–49 years, this may be extended to younger ages if there is evidence of a high risk for CIN2+. HPV detection, VIA and cytology are used for screening (Flowchart 1).

Cervical Cancer Screening Recommendation According to ACOG and ASCCP (2012)

The cervical cancer screening recommendations according to American College of Obstetricians and Gynecologists (ACOG) and American Society for Colposcopy and Cervical Pathology (ASCCP) (2012) are given in Table 2.

Screening should be started regardless of age in HIV positive women or girl, who has started sexual activity. If screening results are negative, women should be rescreened within 3 years. Women treated cervical precancer, should receive post-treatment follow up after 12 months. Screening should continue lifelong.

Table 1: Course of cervical intraepithelial neoplasia (CIN) disease.

CIN type	*Age (years)*	*Regression*	*Persistence*	*Progression*
CIN 1	<30	80–90%	10–20%	1–4%
CIN 2	30–35	30–40%	40%	20%
CIN 3	35–45	20–30%	50–60%	Almost all

Flowchart 1: Cervical cancer screening.

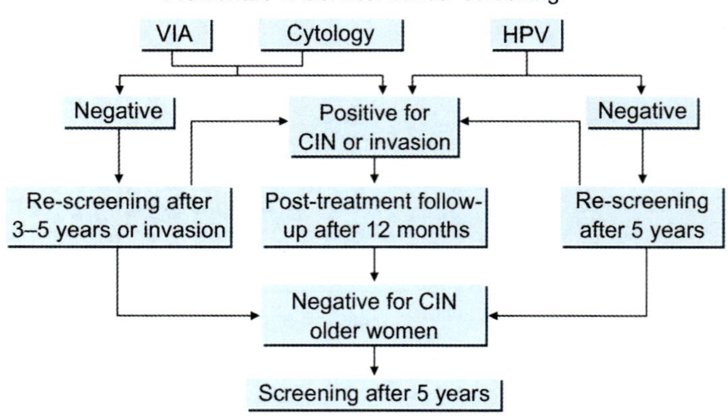

(CIN: cervical intraepithelial neoplasia; HPV: human papilloma virus; VIA: visual inspection with acetic acid)

Table 2: Recommendations of ACOG and ASCCP (2012) for cervical cancer screening.

Patient status	*Recommended screening method*	*Comments*
<21 years old	No screening	Sexual history is not a consideration
21–29 years old	Cytology done every 3 years	
30–65 years old	Preferred—HPV and cytology contesting every 5 years Acceptable—cytology alone every 3 years	
>65 years old	Screening can be discontinue after either 3 consecutive negative cytology test or 2 negative cytology and HPV test within 10 years period, provided the most recent test was within 5 years	Women with a history of CIN 2, CIN3 or adenocarcinoma in situ should continue routine age-based screening for at least 20 years
After total hysterectomy	No screening necessary	Without history of CIN 2, CIN 3, adenocarcinoma in situ or cancer in past 20 years
After supracervical hysterectomy	Routine screening to be followed	
After HPV vaccination	Routine screening to be followed	

Screening during Pregnancy

Pregnancy is not the ideal time to perform screening test. However if a screening test is done and abnormal results are found, the patient should be referred for colposcopy. If colposcopy is not suspicious for invasive cancer, patient should be re-evaluated 6–12 weeks postpartum for colposcopy and possible biopsy if needed.

SCREENING METHODS FOR CERVICAL PRECANCER

Until few years ago, the only method of screening for cervical cancer was Papanicolaou (Pap) smear or cytology. HPV screening tests and visual inspection with acetic acid (VIA) are newer methods for cervical cancer screening in low- and middle-income countries, like India.

HPV Testing

Human papilloma virus testing is highly sensitive for detection for detecting HPV infection in women. Molecular HPV testing methods are based on the detection of DNA from high-risk HPV types in vaginal and/or cervical samples collected by inserting a small brush deep into the vagina. A positive test result in a woman over 30 years age indicates that she may have an existing lesion or may be as risk for future precancer and cancer.

Visual Screening Methods

Visual inspection with acetic acid is a method for detecting early cell changes that are visible when using a speculum to inspect the cervix with naked eye after applying dilute (3–5%) acetic acid to it. *Quite inexpensive, single visit approach* (treatment can be offered at the same visit).

VIA is appropriate to use in women whose squamocolumnar junction is visible. Any acetowhite area which persists even after 1 minute is more likely to be associated with cervical precancer or cancer. It can detect both early changes and those representing more advanced precancers.

Cytology-based Screening Methods

Cytology-based screening involves taking a sample of cells from the entire transformation zone. The cells are either fixed on a slide at the facility (conventional Pap) or placed in a transport medium (liquid-based cytology) and then sent to the laboratory where expert cytotechnologists examine the cells under a microscope. If abnormal cells are seen on microscopic examination, the extent of their abnormality is classified using the Bethesda System.

DIAGNOSTIC TOOLS

These are used on patients with positive screening results to verify the presence, extent and type of precancer or cancer.

Colposcopy

Visualization of cervix, vagina and vulva with an instrument that provides strong light and magnifies a field, allowing specific patterns in the epithelial layer and surrounding blood vessels to be examined. This can be done with a colposcope or especially designed relatively cheap video/digital camera.

Biopsy

Removal of small samples of abnormal tissue for microscopic examination. Biopsy is used to determine the degree of abnormality of the cell changes at the cervix and to rule out cancer. Biopsy to be taken from cancer suspicious areas on the cervix suspected on naked eye, VIA positive or colposcopy examination. In cytology positive cases when lesion not accessible, wedge biopsy, large loop excision of the transformation zone (LLETZ), laser excision or cone biopsy is indicated (Figs. 2 and 3).

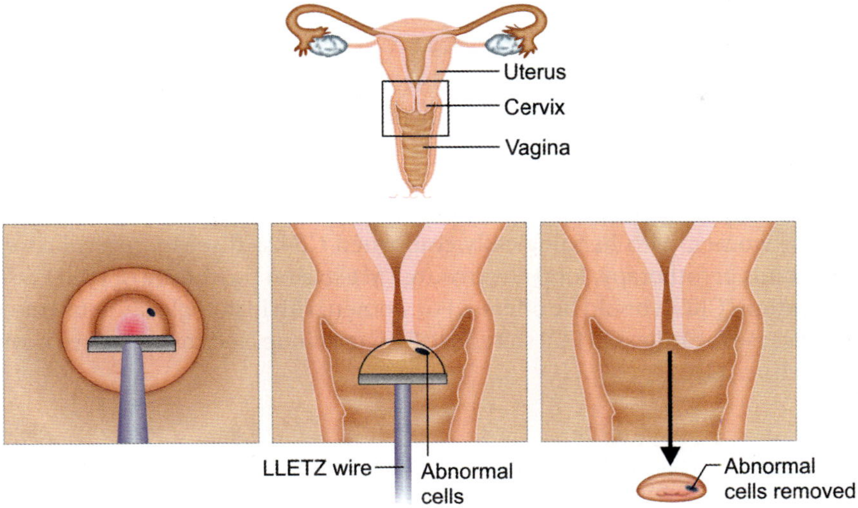

Fig. 2: Large loop excision of the transformation zone (LLETZ).

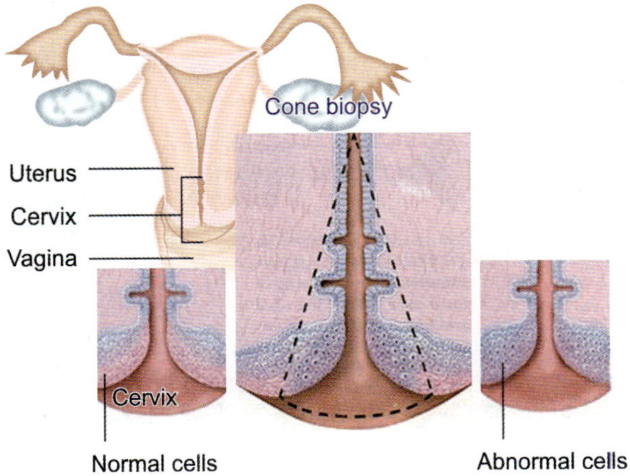

Fig. 3: Cone biopsy.

Endocervical Curettage

Surface cells are gently scraped from the endocervical canal with special thin instrument or spatula, and the tissue is placed in a container with a fixative solution and send to laboratory for examination.

Indications

- Squamocolumnar junction cannot be fully visualized in the face of already suspected lesion.
- Cytology revealed glandular lesion.
- If screening and/or colposcopy were not adequate.

TREATMENT

For cervical cancer prevention to be effective, positive screening must be linked with effective treatment. WHO has considered the two approaches to linking screening and treatment for precancer of the cervix (Flowcharts 2 to 6).

1. Screen, diagnose and treat
2. Screen-and-treat (the single visit approach).

For women with histologically confirmed CIN2+ disease, regardless of HIV status cryotherapy, loop electrosurgical excision procedure or cold knife conization (CKC) should be offered. For women with histologically confirmed AIS disease regardless of HIV status use CKC over loop electrosurgical excision procedure (LEEP).

Flowchart 2: Screen and treat strategies—for screening of cervical cancer using HPV test and VIA.

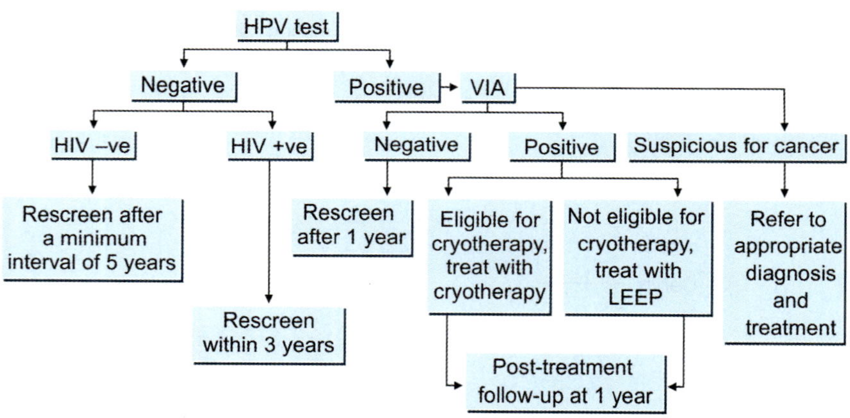

(HIV: human immunodeficiency virus; HPV: human papilloma virus; VIA: visual inspection with acetic acid; LEEP: loop electrosurgical excision procedure)

Flowchart 3: Screen and treat strategies—for screening of cervical cancer using VIA.

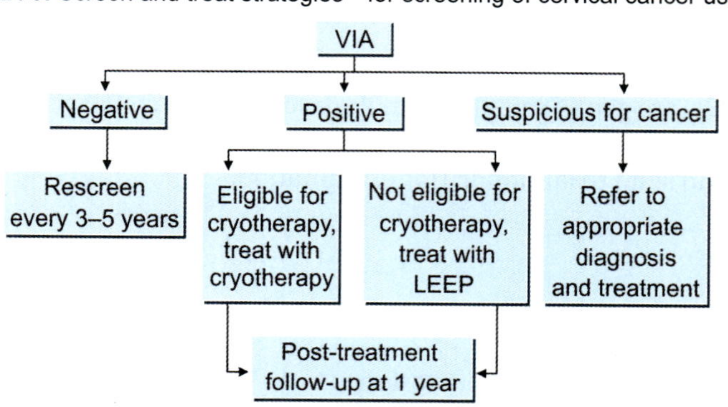

(VIA: visual inspection with acetic acid; LEEP: loop electrosurgical excision procedure)

Flowchart 4: Screen and treat strategies—for screening of cervical cancer using cytology.

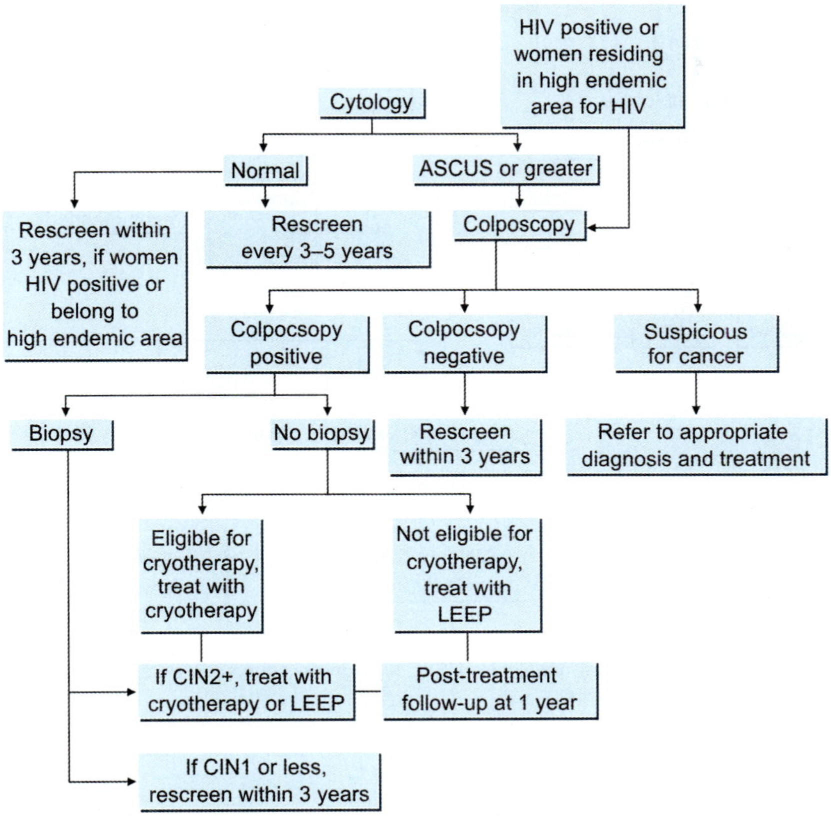

(HIV: human immunodeficiency virus; CIN: cervical intraepithelial neoplasia; LEEP: loop electrosurgical excision procedure; ASCUS: atypical squamous cells of undetermined significance)

Flowchart 5: Management of women with adenocarcinoma in situ diagnosed from diagnostic excisional procedure

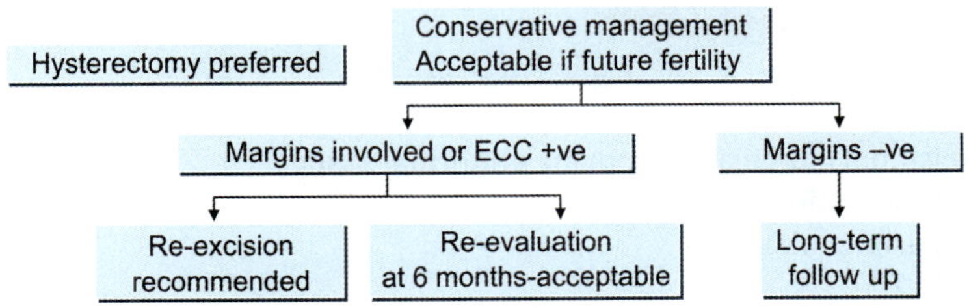

(ECC: endocervical curettage)

Treatment options are (Fig. 4)

- Ablative (destroying abnormal tissue by freezing or burning)
  - Cryotherapy
  - Laser ablation
  - Electrocoagulation

Flowchart 6: Management of adolescent and young women with histological diagnosis of CIN 1.

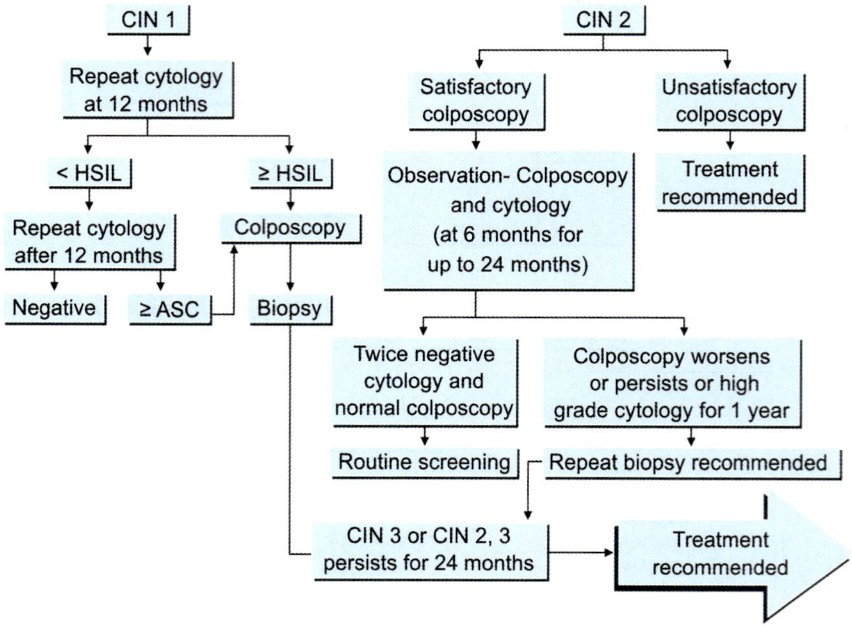

(CIN: cervical intraepithelial neoplasia; HSIL: high-grade squamous intraepithelial lesion; ASC: atypical squamous cells)

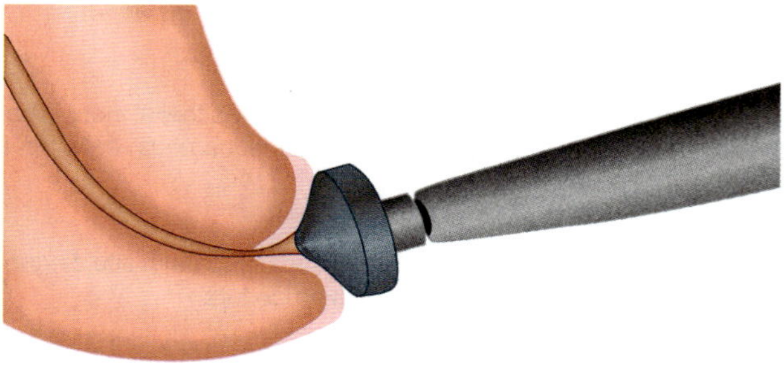

Fig. 4: Laser conization.

- Excisional (surgically removing abnormal tissue)
  - Cold knife conization
  - Laser conization
  - LLETZ
  - LEEP
- Hysterectomy.

Cryotherapy

It eliminates precancerous areas on the cervix by applying cryoprobe to cover the abnormal area over the cervix. The super cooling of the cryoprobe is accomplished using a tank with compressed carbon dioxide (CO_2) or nitrous oxide (N_2O) gas. Following cryotherapy the frozen area regenerates to normal epithelium in a month.

Screen positive or women with histologically confirmed CIN2+ are eligible if

- Entire lesion and SCJ are visible.
- Lesion does not cover more than three-fourths of the ectocervix.

It is contraindicated if lesion is involving endocervix or suspicious of invasive cancer.

Loop Electrosurgical Excision Procedure

It is the removal of abnormal areas from cervix and vagina, using a loop made of thin wire powered by an electrosurgical unit under local anesthesia. The loop tool cuts and coagulates at the same time. This is followed by use of ball electrode to complete the coagulation. It takes 1 month for tissue to regenerate. The SCJ is visible in more than 90% of patients after this procedure.

Screen positive woman or histologically confirmed CIN2+ are eligible, if lesion is not suspicious for invasive cancer.

Cold Knife Conization

Removal of cone-shaped area from the cervix including portions of the ectocervix, whole SCJ and part of endocervix, depending upon size of lesion and likelihood of finding cancer. Tissue removal is sent for the histopathological diagnosis and to ensure that margins are free for complete excision. Usually done in OT under GA or regional anesthesia by surgically trained provider.

It is reserved for cases not fit for ablative or LEEP procedure, and if there is presence of glandular precancer or microinvasion.

Hysterectomy is considered a treatment of last resort for recurrent high-risk CIN.

SUMMARY

As almost all cases of cervical cancer are caused by persistent infection with one or more of the high-risk types of HPV. There are several affordable tests available, which can effectively detect precancer; so that they can be effectively treated with affordable and effective treatment.

FURTHER READING

1. Berek JS. Intraepithelial disease of the cervix, vagina and vulva. In: Berek & Novak's Gynecology 15th edition. Philadelphia: Lippincott Williams & Wilkins; 2012. pp. 1048-99.
2. Hoffman BL, Schorge JO, Schaffer JI, et al. Preinvasive lesions of the lower genital tract. In: Williams Gynecology 2nd edition. New York: McGraw Hill Professional; 2012. pp. 730-56.
3. Karjane N, Chelmow D. New cervical cancer screening guidelines, again. Obs Gynecol Clin. 2013;40(2):211-24.
4. Long S, Leeman L. Treatment option for high-grade squamous intraepithelial lesion. Obstet Gynecol Clin North Am. 2013;40(2):291-316.

5. Massad LS, Einstein MH, Huh WK, et al. 2012 updated consensus guidelines for the management of abnormal cervical cancer screening test and cancer precursors. J Low Genit Tract Dis. 2013;17(5 Suppl 1):S1-S27.
6. Padubidri VG, Daftary SN. Cervical intraepithelial neoplasia, carcinoma of cervix. In: Shaw's Textbook of Gynecology. New Delhi: Reed Elsevier India Private Limited; 2015. pp. 485-94, 498-500.
7. Rock JA, Jones HW III. Cervical cancer precursors and their management. In: Te Linde's Operative Gynecology, 10th edition. Philadelphia: Wolters Kluwer; 2008. pp. 1208-24.
8. World Health Organization. Screening and treatment of cervical pre-cancer. In: Comprehensive cervical cancer control: a guide to essential practice, 2nd edition. Geneva: WHO; 2014. pp. 134-61, 364-73.
9. World Health Organization. WHO guidelines for screening and treatment of precancerous lesion for cervical cancer prevention. Geneva: World Health Organization; 2013.
10. World Health Organization. WHO guidelines for treatment of cervical intraepithelial neoplasia 2–3 and adenocarcinoma in situ. Geneva: World Health Organization; 2014.

Chapter 13

Cryocautery and LLETZ/Leep

Ramani Rajendran

Of recent times, the trend in the treatment of premalignant lesion is toward more conservative approach in which affected area is effectively destroyed.

Irrespective of the modalities used a good preprocedure counseling is mandatory with special stress on the need for continued surveillance for the next 20 years.

TREATMENT OF PREINVASIVE LESION

The purpose of treating precancerous lesions is to destroy the affected areas and thereby reducing the mortality and morbidity associated with cancer cervix.

Cervical intraepithelial neoplasia (CIN) is a premalignant lesion that is diagnosed by histology as CIN1, CIN2, or CIN3. If left untreated, CIN2 or CIN3 (collectively referred to as CIN2+) can progress to cervical cancer.

With regards to CIN1, it is considered as tissue reaction to human papillomavirus (HPV) infection which is transient and there is 60% regression and with low progression rate rises a doubt whether CIN1 should be treated at all.

In low resource countries, see-and-treat policy is advised as the patient compliance is low to follow-up; treatment is the rule of thumb when the lesion persists for 2 years or if the lesion has progressed in size/grade.

The problem with this policy is overtreatment and emotional trauma. But in about 25–40% of women who present with Low-grade squamous intraepithelial lesion (LSIL) on Pap smear can have existing high-grade lesions.

In such cases, reflex HPV DNA testing is test of choice, if the high-risk HPV is not detected, the negative predictive value of this test is almost 99%, conservative management-observation and 6 monthly follow-up is offered. In case high-risk HPV is detected referral to colposcopy is made. A note on biopsy—ideally it should be colpo-directed one and multiple biopsies combined with endocervical curettings if possible for the histopathological confirmation.

Treatment of CIN2 and CIN3 is the ideal option, as this indicates persistent HPV infection and is more likely to progress.

Removal/destruction of the abnormal transformation zone (TZ) is aim of treatment that can of two types.

1. Ablation
2. Excision.

In the ablative procedure, the entire TZ is destroyed in vivo, i.e. no tissue specimen is available for histopathological correlation whereas in the second method the TZ is excised in toto that provides tissue diagnosis.

In the ablative/destructive procedure, three different energy sources are used namely ice in cryocautery heat in thermal coagulation and light in laser vaporization of which cryocautery will be discussed here.

CRYOCAUTERY

Selection Criteria for Ablative Techniques—Cryocautery

- The entire TZ must be visualized, ideally type 1 TZ
- Entire lesion should be on the ectocervix
- Lesion should be adequately covered by the probe
- Lesion should have no endocervical/vaginal extension
- There must be no evidence of glandular abnormality
- Lesion should not occupy more than 75% of the ectocervix
- There must be no evidence of invasive disease
- There must be no previous treatment of cervical precancer lesions
- There must be no discrepancy between cytology, colposcopy and histology.

Exclusion Criteria

- Menstruation
- Pregnancy
- Pelvic inflammatory disease.

Cryocautery Unit

The cryotherapy technique uses a cryoprobe with a tip made of highly conductive metal (usually silver and copper) that makes direct surface contact with the ectocervical lesion (Figs. 1A and B).

A substantial drop in temperature is achieved when a compressed refrigerant gas is allowed to pass through a tiny aperture in the cryoprobe which causes the gas to expand to freezing temperature leading to formation of ice.

Nitrous oxide or carbon dioxide are the refrigerants of choice. Nitrous oxide-based cryotherapy will achieve temperatures of about –89°C and the carbon dioxide-based system will achieve –68°C at the core of the tissue ice ball. The temperature at the edges of the frozen tissue may be around –20°C.

Cells that are frozen at –20°C for 3 minutes will undergo crystallization of the cell water—increase in cell volume—which disrupts the cell membrane leads to cell death, i.e. cryonecrosis.

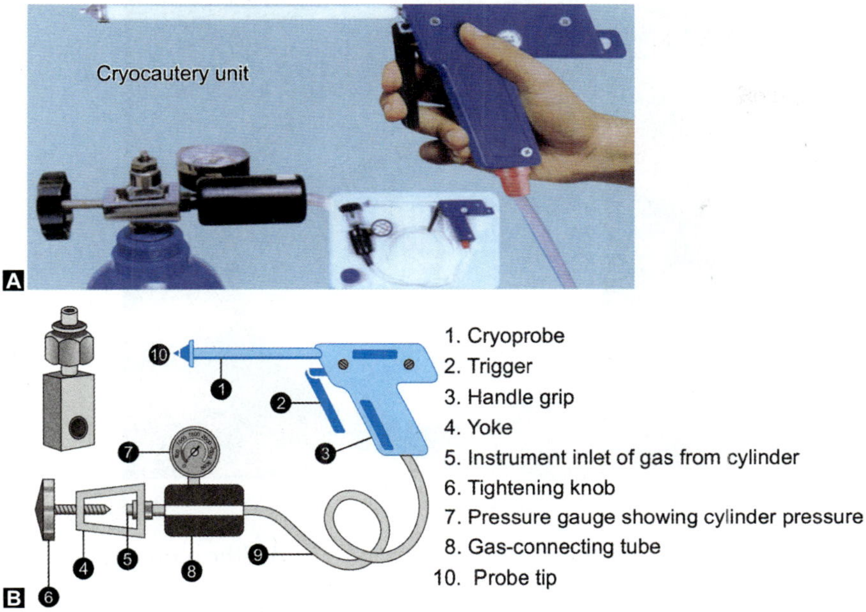

Figs. 1A and B: (A) Cryocautery unit; (B) Cryotherapy equipment and its parts.

Technique

Double-freeze method is used.

Why Double Freeze?

A rapid freeze followed by a slow thaw is the most damaging to cells, a sequence of two freeze-thaw cycles [freeze (3 min)—thaw (5 min), freeze 3 min—thaw (5 min)] may produce more tissue destruction than a single cycle. Depth of destruction is about 4–5 mm.

Steps of Cryocautery

1. Precryocautery counseling (consists of explaining what is cryo, why and how it is done with special mention about the side effects) with informed consent.
2. Check the cryocautery instrument, light source and gas cylinder
   - Once the cylinder is opened to release the gas if the gauge indicator is in the yellow zone indicates low pressure (<40 kg/cm^2), this pressure is insufficient for cryonecrosis so one has to change to a full cylinder.
   - Green zone indicates adequate pressure (40–70 kg/cm^2) and one can proceed to do the procedure (Fig. 2).
3. Under strict aseptic precautions insert the appropriate sized speculum with light source in position so good view of the entire cervix is obtained.
4. Using 5% acetic acid application on the cervix, new squamocolumnar junction (SCJ), TZ is identified and lesion is mapped.

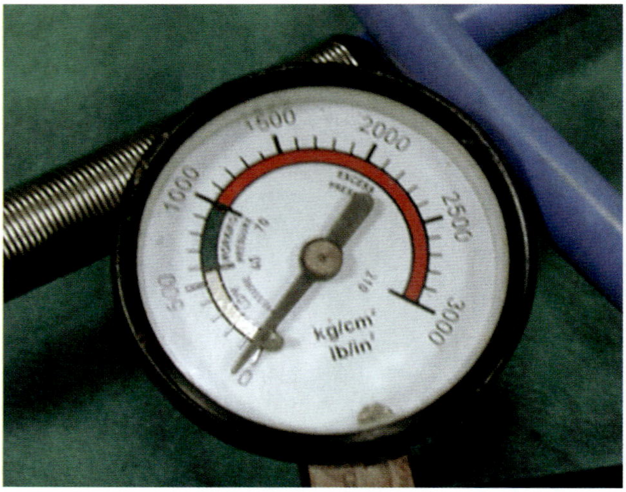

Fig. 2: Gauge indicator.

5. The cryoprobe is coated with lubricant jelly and tip of the probe is placed on the external os of the cervix with precautions to avoid contact with vaginal walls.
6. Trigger of the Cryo-Gun is activated to allow the flow of the gas through shaft to the tip of the probe.
7. Freeze the cervix for 3 minutes ensure the ice ball formation extends 4–5 mm beyond the rim of the cryoprobe.
8. Trigger is released and ice is allowed to thaw for 5 minutes.
9. Repeat the procedure of freezing for another 3 minutes.
10. Once Cryo-Gun is switched off wait for the cryoprobe to detach from the cervix on its own.
11. Remove the probe and speculum one after the other.
12. Decontaminate and sterilize the instruments as mentioned below.

Advantages

- Simple and easy procedure that can be performed with minimal training
- Can be performed without anesthesia
- Safe—no complications
- Single visit approach
- Least expensive equipment
- Needs no electricity
- Cost effective
- Healing is fast
- Fertility is maintained as the endocervical canal is unaltered.

Disadvantages

- No tissue specimen for histopathological examination (HPE)
- Cannot treat lesions with unfavorable size/shape

- Uterine cramping
- Profuse vaginal discharge
- Migration of new SCJ into the endocervix
- Margin status and depth of destruction cannot be gauged correctly so leads to residual lesion.

Post-treatment Instructions

Inform the patient that she will have watery discharge for about 4 weeks which would warrant the use of sanitary pad.

Advice to avoid sexual intercourse for 4 weeks if unavoidable suggested to use condoms.

To report the hospital if she has:

- Fever with chills and rigors
- Foul smelling purulent discharge
- Severe lower abdominal pain/cramps.

Follow-up: The women should return for screening after 1 year.

How to Sterilize the Cryoprobe after Procedure?

- Wash the probe with running water and remove any blood/mucus
- For stubborn stains, use soft brush and soap and again wash with water
- Soak the probe after air drying in 0.1% chlorine solution/2% glutaraldehyde for 20 minutes. Rinse the probe thoroughly with sterile water
- Air dry/dry it with sterile cloth
- Clean the cryoprobe shaft and rest of the cryocautery unit by wiping with cotton soaked in ethyl/isopropyl alcohol.

LARGE LOOP EXCISION OF THE TRANSFORMATION ZONE

This is also referred as loop electrosurgical excision procedure (LEEP). Originally this procedure started off with the use of small loop to obtain biopsy from the cervix. Later on Prendiville et al. have pointed out that when a large loop excision is done it serves a dual purpose of tissue diagnosis and treatment as well. Thus, this procedure gained worldwide popularity. Ease and efficacy of this technique was well documented in both short- and long-term follow-up studies.

Here wire loop electrode powered by the electrosurgical unit is used to remove the entire TZ along the lesion. The electrical heat that is produced by the activated electrode allows excision of the mapped area. A blend of cutting and coagulating current is used for this purpose (Fig. 3).

Principle of Treatment

Large loop excision of the transformation zone (LLETZ) uses monopolar current and therefore needs a ground plate for the electricity to return to the electrosurgical unit after achieving its effect at the point of contact between

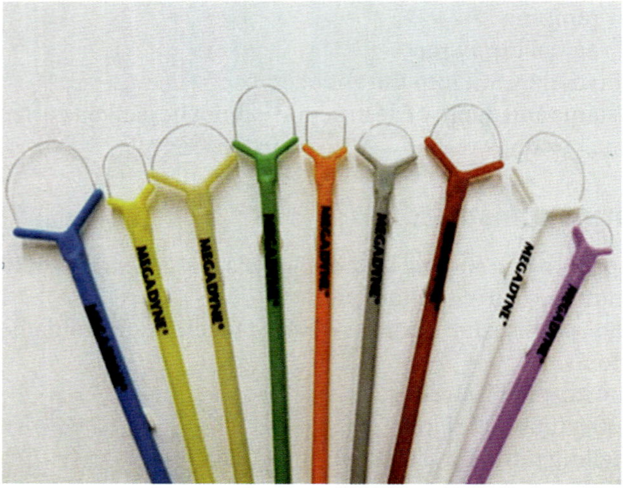

Fig. 3: Loop electrodes of varying sizes and shapes.

the loop and the tissue. Aim is to resect the entire TZ along with a cylindrical block of tissue up to 7 mm thickness.

Different Types of Excision

Type 1 excision: It involves excision of type 1 TZ. This type of excision need not include much of the endocervical canal. Type 1 TZ excision is adequate for CIN2/3 lesions if SCJ is fully visible on the ectocervix.

Type 2 excision: It is indicated if there is CIN2/3 lesion extending to the endocervical canal and when the upper limit of the lesion is clearly visible.

Type 3 excision: It involves excision of type 3 TZ. Here a significant portion of the endocervical canal is excised as the upper limit of the TZ or the lesion is not visible.

Steps of Large Loop Excision of the Transformation Zone

When LLETZ is planned after a thorough counseling with informed consent.

1. Patient is placed on mattress fixed couch with legs placed on the padded stirrup without any metal ornaments/pin/clips on their body for the fear of electrical injury.
2. Return plate is placed in good contact over the buttock.
3. Use of plain stainless steel self-retaining speculum with smoke vent is mandatory (Fig. 4).
   - With time, constant use and cleaning insulated speculum are likely to lose their insulating coat causing current to pass through these bare areas resulting in severe burns.
4. Condom threaded over the speculum helps to keep the lax vaginal walls away.

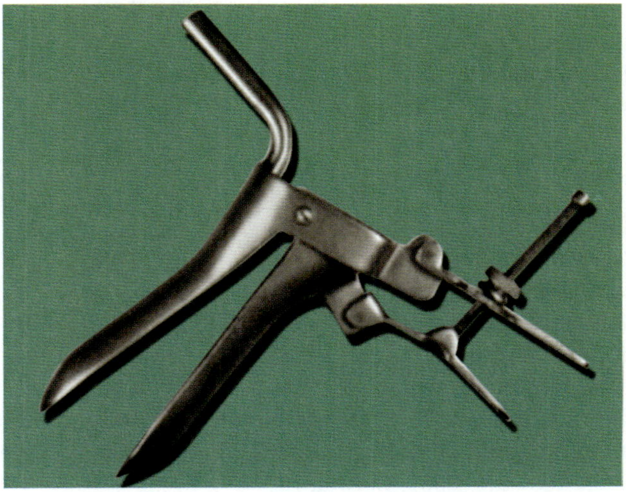

Fig. 4: Plain stainless steel self-retaining speculum with smoke vent.

5. Avoid the use of alcohol-containing fluids, explosive or inflammable fluids when the electrocautery unit is activated.
6. Thorough colposcopic assessment of the cervix, new SCJ and type of TZ 1, 2, 3 is assessed. The lesion is mapped using 5% acetic acid and Lugol's iodine solution.
7. Swede scoring of 8 or more warrants excisional therapy.
8. Local anesthetic—1 mL of 1% lignocaine is injected at 2, 4, 8, 10 o'clock position using dental syringe—such infiltration helps to achieve good hemostasis during the procedure.
9. Connect the suction tubing with vent and switch it on.
10. Fix appropriate size loop to the cautery pen and set the power to blend of 50 watts of coagulation and 50 watts of cutting current.
11. The colposcope is kept at low magnification so that it ensures a panoramic view of the cervix and vagina.
12. Hold inactivated loop few millimeters away from the ectocervix.
13. Later activate the loop by pressing the yellow hand button.
14. Start to pass the loop few millimeters outside the TZ from 9 o'clock position and allow the loop to sink into the substance of the cervix gradually pass it through to exit at other end of TZ at 3 o'clock position.
15. Purpose of this gradual sweep is to get the entire TZ with the lesion as a single piece with good hemostasis—the specimen is marked and fixed immediately with formalin on cork board.
16. Hemostasis is achieved either by application of Monsel's paste/fulgurating the base of the crater with small ball diathermy.
17. Document the procedure.
18. Postprocedure counsel about abstinence for 4–6 weeks and the presence of pink watery discharge with mild discomfort.

19. Stress on the need to report to the hospital if there is severe bleeding with lower abdominal pain.
20. Emphasize on the visit to the hospital for collection of HPE report and to discuss about the follow-up plan.

Advantages

- Treatment time is shorter
- Easier to learn
- No hazard to the eyes unlike laser
- Equipment less costly
- Less handling of tissues
- Sample tissue is better than laser.

Gained popularity as efficacy was well documented in both short- and long-term follow-up studies (Prendiville 1989, Bigrigg 1990, Whiteley and Olah 1990, Flannelly 1997 and 2001, Gardial 1997).

Disadvantages

Long-term cervical morphological change that leads to:
- Stenosis—dysmenorrhea
- Cervical incompetence—pregnancy complications—miscarriage and premature labor.

Histopathological examination report: Specimen should be removed as a single sample.
Removal in multiple fragments leads to:
- Difficulty histopathological assessment
- Difficulty to allocate a substage
- Delineate completeness of excision.

Apart from the pathological diagnosis of the lesion, the most important feature is to note the status of excised margins. Those with positive disease margins especially at the endocervical resected end are more prone recurrent disease.

Follow-Up Plan

Follow-up is essential as there is less than 10% chance of having residual disease which could progress to cancer. This increased risk lasts for next 20 years.

Women aged 50 years or older are particularly at high risk of persistent/recurrent disease.

Human papillomavirus testing is the most sensitive and accurate test to detect residual/recurrent disease. It has the best negative predictive value but the only disadvantage being its high cost. Irrespective of the available and affordable modalites those treated of precancerous lesions need to be followed for the next 20 years.

Chapter 14

Prophylactic Salpingectomy at Hysterectomy for Benign Diseases as an Effective Tool for Reducing Pelvic Serous Carcinoma: A Prospective Case Control Study

Tushar Kar, Asaranti Kar, Bhagyalaxmi Nayak, Ipsita Dhal

INTRODUCTION

Pelvic high-grade serous carcinomas (HGSCs), including ovarian carcinoma (OC), tubal carcinoma (TC), and primary peritoneal carcinomas (PPC), receive much attention from clinicians and researchers because of their usually advanced stage at presentation, rapid progression, extraovarian disease at the time of diagnosis, poor prognosis and high fatality rate. Lack of a proper screening method in these cases is the cause of their late detection. Recently, the distal fallopian tube has been documented as a common (80%) site of tumor origin in BRCA+ve (BRCA1 or BRCA2) women undergoing risk reducing salpingo-oophorectomy.[1,2] Also it has been demonstrated in a series of unselected women with pelvic serous carcinoma that serous tubal intraepithelial carcinoma (STIC) may precede a significant percentage of these tumors.

Salpingectomy at the time of hysterectomy or during tubal sterilization, compared with hysterectomy alone or tubal ligation can be considered safe and without an increase in complications or readmissions.[3] Also, based on surrogate serum markers or response to in vitro fertilization, ovarian function does not get affected by salpingectomy at the time of hysterectomy.[4-7] On the contrary, when patients undergo an operation during which the fallopian tubes could be removed in addition to the primary surgical procedure like hysterectomy, the risk of ovarian cancer may be further reduced. Therefore, ovarian conservation and salpingectomy may be considered a better option than bilateral salpingo-oophorectomy for ovarian cancer risk reduction in women undergoing other pelvic surgeries for benign diseases. But the value of salpingectomy at benign hysterectomy remains to be determined with certainty.[8]

Given the complexities involved about the origin of pelvic serous cancers it is important to investigate the roles of fallopian tubes with regard to the occurrence of p53 signature, tubal intraepithelial lesions in transition (TILT) and STIC. So, in this project we studied the association of tubal precancerous lesions in a consecutive series of sporadic OC, TC and PPC and controls comprising of low grade OC and benign adnexal masses.

MATERIAL AND METHODS

The study was carried out in Department of Obstetrics and Gynaecology, Department of Pathology and Department of Oncopathology within a period of 2 years. A group of control patients were taken which included benign ovarian adnexal masses and low grade ovarian tumors.

All histopathologically diagnosed cases of pelvic high-grade serous carcinoma were considered as the study group. Both sides of fallopian tubes were grossed according to "SEE-FIM" protocol (sectioning and extensively examining the fimbriated end).[9] By this method, multiple longitudinal sections of the distal two cm of the tube were taken (usually 2–3 sections). Serial transverse sections (every 2–3 mm) were taken from the isthmus and ampulla (6–8 sections). The sections were examined histopathologically and immunohistochemically for p53 and Ki67 for detection of various precursor lesions. The results of histopathology and immunohistochemistry were noted down in tabulated manner. The paired t-test and one way ANOVA were employed to find out the correlation between desired variables. The result was considered statistically significant if p value was less than 0.05.

For morphological analysis of different steps in serous carcinogenesis in fallopian tube, the histopathological and immunohistochemical features are put forth by Lee et al. and Crum et al.[10,11] Diagnostic algorithm proposed by Vang et al was utilized for the diagnosis of precursor lesions incorporating results of morphology and immunohistochemical findings.[12] p53 signature is characterised by low proliferative index (<10% nuclei positive for Ki67) with mild cytologic atypia and secretory cell outgrowth. p53 immunostaining shows accumulation of p53 in linear stretch of 12 or more consecutive secretory cell nuclei. STIC is diagnosed by stratification of secretory cells, loss of polarity, architectural distortion, atypia and strong staining of many nuclei with p53 and high proliferative index (>10% nuclei positive for Ki67). TILT is the intermediate lesion with features in between the above two extreme conditions.

RESULTS

Total 86 cases were included in the study, out of which 55 cases belonged to pelvic human genome sequencing center (HGSC) categorized into different groups based on the conventional criteria of diagnosis as devised by WHO.[13,14]

Accordingly, they were classified into ovarian (50 or 90.9% cases), PPC (3 or 5.5% cases) and tubal (2 or 3.6% cases) Control group included 21 cases (26% of total ovarian masses) of low-grade serous carcinoma (LGSC) of ovary and 10 cases (12%) of benign adnexal masses (non-neoplastic ovarian cysts). Age of the patients ranged from 29 years to 72 years; mean ± SD was 47 ± 9.89 years. Majority were detected in 4th decades of life (36%). Predominantly the patients were of parity 2 (20 cases, 36%), followed by P1 in 13 cases (23.6%), least number of cases was nullipara (7%) (Table 1). Out of them, 32 (58.1%) were premenopausal and 23 (41.9%) were postmenopausal (p value was non-significant = 0.579). Family history of pelvic carcinoma was present in 29 cases (53%).

Twenty-seven patients had ascites at the time of presentation, out of which malignant cells were found in 5 cases (majority being ovarian-4 cases) and 21 (38%) had omental deposits from which 17 cases (80.95%) belonged to ovarian

Table 1: Characteristics of ovarian, peritoneal and tubal high-grade serous carcinoma.

Factor	*Ovarian*	*Tubal*	*Peritoneal*	*Total*
Parity 0	4	0	0	4 (7.27%)
Parity 1	13	0	0	13 (23.6%)
Parity 2	17	1	2	20 (36.3%)
Parity 3	9	2	0	11 (20%)
Parity 4	5	0	0	5 (9.09%)
Premenopausal	31	0	1	32 (58.18%)
Postmenopausal	19	3	1	23 (41.82%)
Presence of ascites	24	2	1	27 (49.09%)
Malignant cells in ascitic fluid	4	0	1	5 (9.09%)
Omental deposits present	17	2	2	21 (38%)
Size of tumor ≤4 cm	11	1	2	14(25.4%)
Size of tumor>4 ≤8 cm	36	3	2	38(69.2%)
Size of tumor >8 cm	3	0	0	3 (5.4%)
Mostly solid in consistency	25	2	2	29 (53%)
Mostly cystic in consistency	9	0	0	9 (16%)
Mixed consistency	16	1	0	17 (31%)
FIGO stage I tumors	6	0	0	6 (11%)
FIGO stage II tumors	15	2	1	18 (33%)
FIGO stage III tumors	16	1	1	18 (33%)
FIGO stage IV tumors	13	0	0	13 (23%)
Occurrence of p53 signature	13	0	1	14 (25.45%)
Occurrence of TILT	10	0	0	10(18.18%)
Occurrence of STIC	14	1	1	16 (29.09%)

HGSC. Most common size was between 4 cm and 6 cm, mean ± SD was 4.97 ± 1.52 cm (*p* value was significant = 0.0329). Most of the women (36 = 66%) were in stage II and III (p value was 0.0002 = extremely significant) (Table 1). In the present study, majority of the tumors (29 cases,53%) were predominantly solid and least were predominantly cystic in consistency (9 cases 16%). High-grade pelvic tumors mostly belonged to FIGO stage II and III (36 cases, 66%) with least number of cases (6 cases or 11%) in stage I. Ovarian tumors were mostly of stage III (16 cases), followed by stage II (15 cases), stage IV (13 cases) and stage I (6 cases), respectively. Out of the 3 cases of tubal carcinoma, 2 were of stage II and out of the 2 cases of PPC one each was of stage II and stage III. One way ANOVA, p value was found to be 0.0002 which was extremely significant.

Evidence of various precursor lesions in fallopian tube was detected in 40 cases (72.72%). Precursor lesions like p53 signature, TILT and STIC were most commonly encountered in OHGSC (37/55 cases, 67.27%) (Table 2). The predominant tubal intraepithelial lesion was STIC; seen in 16/55 cases (29.09%). Out of 50 cases of OHGSC, 13 cases showed p53 signature (26%), 10 (20%) showed TILT and 14 cases (28%) were STIC positive with significant p value (0.0474). Both cases of tubal serous carcinoma had shown presence of STIC. And out of primary peritoneal serous carcinoma, one case each had presence of p53 signature and STIC in one side tube. But none of the control cases showed positivity for any precursor lesions.

DISCUSSION

Salpingectomy is a prophylactic or preventive surgery to remove the entire fallopian tubes with all hysterectomies for women at high risk of ovarian,

Table 2: Distribution of precursor lesions in different groups.

	Precursor lesions / *Ovarian lesions*	*Number of cases studied*	*'P53 signature' +ve cases (%)*	*TILT +ve cases (%)*	*STIC +ve cases (%)*
CASES	Pelvic high-grade papillary serous carcinoma	50	13 (26%)	10 (20%)	14 (28%)
CONTROLS	Low-grade papillary serous carcinoma	10	0 (0%)	0 (0%)	0 (0%)
	Benign cysts of ovary	21	0 (0%)	0 (0%)	0 (0%)
	Benign				

tubal and peritoneal cancers. For last few decades, the fallopian tube is being targeted as a future method of prevention of such malignancies since screening and early detection are unsuccessful. It has been suggested that one-third to nearly half of pelvic serous carcinomas have presence of tubal intraepithelial carcinoma in association. This leads to the belief that a subset of carcinomas which appear to be primary ovarian or peritoneal HGSCs may be of fallopian tube origin besides the invasive tubal carcinoma which arise from tubal intramucosal carcinoma. In women with a genetic predisposition for ovarian cancer, lesions have been found in the fallopian tubes that closely resemble ovarian HGSC or STIC. These lesions are thought to be the primary source of ovarian carcinoma that secondarily involves the ovary. Manchanda R et al. in a study found that both high-risk women of unknown mutation status and BRCA carriers have a significant (1.05% and 5.1% respectively) rate of occult invasive/in situ tubal/ovarian cancer.[15]

Hence, prophylactic salpingectomy may offer clinicians the opportunity to prevent ovarian cancer in their patients. Between 1 in 400 and 1 in 800 people in the US population carry one of the causative mutations, and salpingectomy has become the standard management. This has resulted in marginal improvement of overall survival rate for women with epithelial ovarian cancer in the past 50 years. Therefore in the present study, we have tried to document presence of precursor lesions of pelvic serous carcinoma, i.e. STIC, TILT and p53 signature in a series of consecutive cases of ovarian, tubal and peritoneal carcinomas. This study was conducted on 55 consecutive cases of high-grade pelvic serous carcinoma along with 21 low-grade ovarian serous carcinoma and 10 benign ovarian cysts. Mittal N et al.[16] studied 32 high grade pelvic serous carcinoma and found ovarian in 62.5% cases, tubal in 6.25% of cases, and peritoneal in 31.25% of cases as per existing criteria of WHO. In comparison there are increased incidences of ovarian HGSC in this series which needs further studies to establish it and also rigorous screening, prophylaxis and management protocols are necessary to reduce this high incidence in this region.

Out of 50 cases of ovarian HGSC, 13 (26%) showed p53 signature, 10 (20%) had TILT positivity and 14 (28%) were STIC positive. Tang S et al. had detected STIC in 6 out of 32 cases of HGSC of ovary and 2 out of 7 cases of PPC.[17] Kindelberger DW et al. detected STIC in 29 of 41 (71%) cases of pelvic serous carcinoma.[18] This is comparable with our data as in present study precursor lesions were seen in 40 of 55 cases (72%). Tubal p53 signature was observed in 29 out of 75 (38%) cases of HGSC of ovary which is similar to our findings (26%). Above study showed p53 signature, TILT and STIC in 26%, 20% and 28% in HGSC, 50%, 0% and 50% in TC and 0%, 0% and 33% in PPC, respectively. This observation is well supported by Leonhardt K et al. where frequency of p53 signature, TILT and STIC were 35.7%, 7.1% and 0% in cases of prophylactic BSO, 18.2%. 9.1% and 18.2% in TC and 11.1%, 0% and 33.3% in PPC.[19] STIC was seen only in fimbrial end of tube which is supported by Mittal N et al. who also got in all cases STIC.[16] Kindelberger et al. and Przybycin CG et al. got STIC in fimbrial end in 92–93% of patients.[18,20]

CONCLUSION

Based on the results of this study and of multiple other studies reported in the literature, it can be concluded that, TIC acts as a precursor lesion for most of the ovarian, fallopian tube, and primary peritoneal HGSCs. Their similar histogenesis has led to a common staging system in all the pelvic carcinomas (FIGO, Rome 2012).[21] Thus prophylactic salpingectomy while performing hysterectomy and doing fimbriectomy as opposed to tubal ligation for tubal sterilization can be adopted as a screening and preventive method for these lethal entities. These initiatives have already been taken at some places of the world, like Vancouver General Hospital and British Columbia Cancer Agency;[12] however, future clinical trials are necessary.

By knowing the real culprit for the carcinogenesis of these tumors we can achieve ultimate goal of reduction in incidence and down-staging of pelvic serous carcinomas. Therefore, extremely thorough histopathological examination of the fimbriated end of the fallopian tubes in all cases of adnexal masses is mandatory to look for any precursor lesions.

REFERENCES

1. Crum CP. Intercepting pelvic cancer in the distal fallopian tube: theories and realities. Mol Oncol. 2009;3:165-70.
2. Herrington CS, Mc Cluggage WG. The emerging role of the distal Fallopian tube and p53 in pelvic serous carcinogenesis. J Pathol. 2010;220:5-6.
3. McAlpine JN, Hanley GE, Woo MM, et al. Opportunistic salpingectomy: uptake, risks, and complications of a regional initiative for ovarian cancer prevention. Ovarian Cancer Research Program of British Columbia. Am J Obstet Gynecol. 2014;210:471.e1-11.
4. Findley AD, Siedhoff MT, Hobbs KA, et al. Short-term effects of salpingectomy during laparoscopic hysterectomy on ovarian reserve: a pilot randomized controlled trial. Fertil Steril. 2013;100:1704-8.
5. Sezik M, Ozkaya O, Demir F, et al. Total salpingectomy during abdominal hysterectomy: effects on ovarian reserve and ovarian stromal blood flow. J Obstet Gynaecol Res. 2007;33:863-9.
6. Morelli M, Venturella R, Mocciaro R, et al. Prophylactic salpingectomy in premenopausal low-risk women for ovarian cancer: primum non nocere. Gynecol Oncol. 2013;129:448-51.
7. Almog B, Wagman I, Bibi G, et al. Effects of salpingectomy on ovarian response in controlled ovarian hyperstimulation for in vitro fertilization: a reappraisal. Fertil Steril. 2011;95:2474-6.
8. Anderson CK, Wallace S, Guiahi M, et al. Risk-reducing salpingectomy as preventive strategy for pelvic serous cancers. Int J Gynecol Cancer. 2013;23:417-21.
9. Medeiros F, Muto MG, Lee Y, et al. The tubal fimbria is a preferred site for early adenocarcinoma in women with familial ovarian cancer syndrome. Am J Surg Pathol. 2006;30:230-6.
10. Lee Y, Miron A, Drapkin R, et al. A candidate precursor to serous carcinoma that originates in the distal fallopian tube. J Pathol. 2007, 211:26-35.
11. Crum CP, Drapkin R, Kindelberger D, et al. Lessons from BRCA: the tubal fimbria emerges as an origin for pelvic serous cancer. Clin Med Res. 2007;5:35-44.
12. Vang R, Shih I, Kurman RJ. Fallopian tube precursors of ovarian low- and high-grade serous neoplasms. J of Histopathology. 2013,62:44-58.
13. Benedet JL, Ngan HYS, Hacker NF. For the FIGO committee on Gynecologic Oncology. Staging classifications and clinical practice guidelines of gynecologic cancers. Int J Gynecol Obstet. 2000;70:209-62.
14. Lee KR, Tavassoli FA, Prat J, et al. Surface epithelial–stromal tumors. In: Tavassoli FA, Deville P (Eds.) World Health Organization classification of tumors. Pathology and genetics of tumors of the breast and female genital organs. Lyon, France: IARC Press; 2003.p117-45.

15. Manchanda R, Silvanto A, Abdelraheim A, et al. Diathermy induced injury may affect detection of occult tubal lesions at risk-reducing salpingo-oophorectomy. Int J Gynecol Cancer. 2012 Jun;22(5):881-8.
16. Mittal N, Srinivasan R, Gupta N, et al. Secretory cell outgrowths, p53 signatures, and serous tubal intraepithelial carcinoma in the fallopian tubes of patients with sporadic pelvic serous carcinoma. Indian J Pathol Microbiol. 2016;59:481-8.
17. Tang S, Onuma K, Deb P, et al. Frequency of Serous Tubal Intraepithelial Carcinoma in Various Gynecologic Malignancies: A Study of 300 Consecutive Cases. Int J Gynecol Pathol. 2012;31(2):103-10.
18. Kindelberger DW, Lee Y, Miron A, et al. Intraepithelial carcinoma of the fimbria and pelvic serous carcinoma: evidence for a causal relationship. Am J Surg Pathol. 2007;31:161-9.
19. Leonhardt K, Einenkel J, Sohr S, et al. p53 signature and serous tubal in-situ carcinoma in cases of primary tubal and peritoneal carcinomas and serous borderline tumors of the ovary. Int J Gynecol Pathol. 2011;30:417-24.
20. Przybycin CG, Kurman RJ, Ronnett BM, et al. Are all pelvic (nonuterine) serous carcinomas of tubal origin? Am J Surg Pathol. 2010;34:1407-16.
21. Jaime P and FIGO Committee on Gynecological Oncology. FIGO's staging classification for cancer of ovary, fallopian tube and peritoneum: abridged republication. J Gynecol Oncol. 2015;26:87-9.